Respect-Focused Therapy

T0386606

"It's rare to find a new, emerging approach so comprehensive and concrete. This represents a dynamic move forward for the mental health and social service field."
—**Gena M. Minnix**, *Seminary of the Southwest, TX*

"With a sound theoretical base in familiar developmental and psychological theory, Slay-Westbrook offers a unique framework for clinicians that makes respect a centerpiece of the therapeutic process and highlights the importance of respect as a focus in helping to heal damage done by its absence."
—**Diane M. Harvey**, *Licensed Clinical Social Worker, TX*

Therapists have a unique opportunity and responsibility to provide a respectful environment for their clients, yet respect has not received adequate attention in the psychotherapy community and related research. *Respect-Focused Therapy: Honoring Clients Through the Therapeutic Relationship and Process* sets forth the formulation of respect-focused therapy (RFT), a new approach to psychotherapy that addresses the quality of the client–therapist relationship. This volume treats respect as a combination of action, attitude and open-mindedness, urging therapists to recognize their own biases and beliefs and be willing to suspend them for the benefit of their clients. Using Martin Buber's "I-Thou" relationship as a conceptual model, Slay-Westbrook provides core principles of respect and demonstrates how to incorporate these into the therapeutic relationship to best foster a healing environment.

Susanne Slay-Westbrook is a practicing professional counselor and marriage and family therapist in Texas, US.

Explorations in Mental Health Series

For a full list of titles in this series, please visit www.routledge.com

Respect-Focused Therapy

Honoring Clients Through
the Therapeutic Relationship
and Process

Susanne Slay-Westbrook

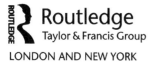

Routledge
Taylor & Francis Group

LONDON AND NEW YORK

First published 2017 by Routledge

2 Park Square, Milton Park, Abingdon, Oxfordshire OX14 4RN
52 Vanderbilt Avenue, New York, NY 10017

Routledge is an imprint of the Taylor & Francis Group, an informa business

First issued in paperback 2018

Library of Congress Cataloguing-in-Publication Data
Names: Slay-Westbrook, Susanne, author.
Title: Respect-focused therapy : honoring clients through the
    therapeutic relationship and process / by Susanne Slay-Westbrook.
Other titles: Explorations in mental health series.
Description: New York : Routledge, 2017. | Series: Explorations
    in mental health series | Includes bibliographical references.
Identifiers: LCCN 2016021378 | ISBN 9781138906907 (hbk) |
    ISBN 9781315695303 (ebk)
Subjects: MESH: Psychotherapy—methods | Social Behavior |
    Physician-Patient Relations | Interpersonal Relations | Case Reports
Classification: LCC RC480.5 | NLM WM 420 | DDC 616.89/14—dc23
LC record available at https://lccn.loc.gov/2016021378

ISBN: 978-1-138-90690-7 (hbk)
ISBN: 978-0-367-19610-3 (pbk)

Typeset in Sabon
by Apex CoVantage, LLC

To my parents
Ruth and Cooper Slay

Contents

Figures

Foreword

Susanne Slay-Westbrook breathes life into the notion of respect by showing that when deeply understood, it involves far more than civility and good manners. From this viewpoint, respect means engaging with others in an attitude of openness and connecting with and wholeheartedly valuing the particular person who is in front of oneself. As one engages with the other in this way, a dynamic process of caring comes into being. When the relationship continues and endures, healing becomes increasingly possible.

I have worked and taught in the field of mental health and psychology for close to 50 years, and I am convinced that we do not need one more book or manual that promises a new method for bringing about miraculous transformations in psychotherapy. Instead, by emphasizing the critical role that a respectful attitude plays in psychotherapy, as well as in other relationships, the author takes us into the realm of already existing human possibilities, possibilities that are present in any human interaction, however much we may habitually overlook them. Her book does not minimize human suffering and tragedy. Rather, through examples of her work with clients, many of whom have experienced powerful trauma as well as neglect, she shows us concretely what a respectful approach looks like. She shows how it can quietly and slowly infuse a sense of hope into the lives of clients who have been treated with disrespect for years and years. It is one thing for clients (or anyone) to realize that they are not alone with their pain and distress; it adds another layer when they see that the person who is listening (be it a therapist or friend or family member) listens with appreciation and attentiveness to oneself as a unique person, that is, with respect.

This is not an encounter with something abstract but something that is immediate and viscerally felt and memorable. Experiencing respect is certainly of great value to the person who is being helped, but it is also uplifting and life giving for the person who is helping. There is, in such a relationship, a process of giving and receiving; in respecting the other, we become more human ourselves, sometimes even surprising ourselves by the extent of the caring that arises within us.

In this context, Slay-Westbrook rightly discusses the contributions of the existential philosopher Martin Buber. Buber has added much to our understanding of human interactions and the ethical dimension that is always implicitly at work in them. He has written extensively of the I-Thou relationship, a term he uses to characterize a relationship when two people encounter each other in a radically open and mutual way and where each person is present and available to the other. In this relationship we grow as persons, or as he would say, become more fully human. Respect for the other is at the core of the I-Thou relationship, and although therapy relationships are ordinarily not mutual in nature (one person is seeking help from another), the respect of the therapist for the client gradually enables that person to develop respect and appreciation for the self, eventually allowing for the possibility of mutuality as therapy comes to the end.

Susanne Slay-Westbrook brings to the writing of this book 40 years of experience as a psychotherapist, couples and family counselor, and supervisor of counselors. Moreover, as a person with cerebral palsy, she has encountered far more than her share of lack of respect for her abilities and potential. I met Susanne when she was a psychology major at Seton Hill University in Pennsylvania back in the mid-1970s. As a faculty member I was impressed with the quality of her academic work, and with her commitment and determination to grow intellectually and professionally, as well as her kindness and caring attitude. In reading her book I have been moved by her accounts of therapeutic work with a wide range of individuals, couples, and families. For Susanne, respect is not a slogan but an attitude that she has embodied over the years. Her reflections on this fundamental approach to relationships and to psychotherapy have given rise to new insights into the healing relationship. Just as significantly, what she says in this book is affirming of what we as psychotherapists and counselors who value the relational dimension of therapy have always known, even if we did not quite have words for it: It is the deep and unsentimental appreciation for clients and the continuing willingness to take a second look at who the other really is beyond our preconceptions and biases that provide the foundation and energy for our vocation.

As Susanne states in her conclusion, "the root of the word 'respectare' or 'respicere' means literally to look back or to reconsider." I think all of us can readily think of times in our personal or professional relationships when we came to take a second look at someone we thought we knew very well and then saw that person as if for the first time. These moments bring new life to our relationships, and sometimes they may even salvage relationships that seemed to be falling apart or have no future. Similarly, we cherish those moments when we felt really seen and respected by another person. Susanne addresses these fundamental realities as well as the nature of psychotherapy in a way that is original, compelling, and persuasive.

Steen Halling
Professor Emeritus
Seattle University

Preface

I've had the great honor of being a mental health professional for almost 40 years. About 20 years ago I was asked to be a part of a panel on a radio show about gangs. I had recently attended several workshops and conferences on that topic and felt reasonably prepared to serve as an "expert" on the subject. To my surprise, there were some real gang members as well as other experts present. I was a bit rattled, but I was a professional after all and felt confident in my competency. All was going well for about 10 minutes, but as I listened to the gang members continue to speak, I kept hearing a word I didn't understand and had never heard of before: "Dissed." What in the world is "dissed?" I had no idea, nor did I know how to respond. Needless to say, I kept pretty quiet through most of the interview and listened. I was ever so grateful that I did because I learned so much that I eventually refocused the entire approach to my therapy practice.

The word, of course, means to be disrespected. I was trying to figure this out as they spoke. I was moved by how passionately they spoke about it. They expressed so much pain and anger around this word. It was a bark and a cry at the same time. It became clear that this was a central theme in their lives. I never learned the history of their life experiences, but I was confident they were pretty shattering. What made me even sadder was the realization that their collective response to being disrespected was to demand it with the force of weapons, which probably never got them what they were really looking for.

At the time, I was also writing a weekly mental health column called *The Coping Corner* in a local Houston newspaper. Because it was weekly, I was forever trying to drum up new topics to write about, and hence I wrote a series of columns about respect. As I continued down this path, two things surprised me. First, I found little to no research material on this topic—largely true still today—and second, the more I thought about it, the more relevant material I realized there was to write about.

Outgrowing the containment of my column, I spilled into writing my first book, *A World of Respect,* published in 2001. In that book I wrote about respect in a broader sense, the lost art of respect in our society and the need to regrow and nurture it within ourselves and in our relationships, families, communities, and globally. This book was published just after 9/11, which put a huge exclamation mark on the relevancy of it for me.

Much has changed since then. Of greatest note, two extended wars and contentious religious and political conflicts are flaring and brewing all over the world. From 9/11 forward, it seems that hatred, division, territorialism, greed, and power have only escalated and play a very ugly part in our lives. Violence continues not only abroad but in this hemisphere as well. Mass shootings at schools and shopping malls, gang activity, and family violence are just some examples. There are so many examples of horrific discord offered to us by the nightly news that we feel helpless against it and become numb to it instead.

Therapists, however, do have a greater opportunity to help implement change on a more personal level. Working directly with individuals, couples, families, and groups, we have the honor of intersecting people's lives in a way that few other professionals do. They come bearing their most private emotional pain, asking us to help them find their way out of that pain. This creates for us an enormous responsibility but also an equal amount of power, each of which we often underestimate. We go to many training sessions, conferences, and ethics workshops, but I believe we frequently miss the most critical piece in the wider scope of our work, which is the actual relationship we have with our client.

When I talk to colleagues about respect, at least initially, I often get back a curious but confused look. Trying to understand this response, I gather two things are going on. First, I think that the word itself is misunderstood and thereby undervalued. Many I believe hear the word and think, "Respect your elders or authority," or even more simply, "Have good manners." Whereas the meaning may well include these notions, it encompasses much more depth and quality.

The Latin root, *respectare*, means "to look back, to look again, or to reconsider." This gives this word more richness and complexity. It is no longer about reflexive, politically appropriate responses to social circumstances but a much greater, more genuine willingness to hear and try to understand and appreciate, even if we disagree. It is at this level that I think respect is frequently missed in meaning and in deed.

Second, and sadly ironic, I fear that many of my colleagues may feel a bit disrespected by the very idea that I suggest respect is underrepresented in our work. This is not meant to minimize the tremendous skill and dedication we each bring to our profession, nor do I mean to say that any of us purposely choose not to bring respect into the therapy room. I do believe that for all of us, respect can become an elusive and presumed part of the process that inadvertently gets overlooked. We're all human, and we come with our own biases and preconceptions that often sit in the background of our consciousness so that they may go without our notice unless we are purposefully aware.

The value in this discussion is to celebrate all of who we are, including our flaws, and find new ways to help our clients do the same. The more awareness and acceptance we have of our own humanness, the more we can be available to do the same for others. I'm convinced this isn't a one-time "ah-ha" moment in which we reach this awareness rather an ongoing struggle from within to transcend and move beyond our own previous limitations. It is from within, the acceptance of who we really are, that gives us the grace to be able to change for the better.

One personal point of disclosure that I choose to include in this discussion is the fact that I have a visible physical disability, cerebral palsy (CP), which functionally means that I use a power wheelchair for mobility. I bring this up to recognize some of my more obvious imperfections as well as to point to my experience with social disrespect over a lifetime. Persons with CP, and other disabilities, have been historically stereotyped as being mentally and/or spiritually deficient, both of which deeply undermine the value and potential of such persons. When I was in graduate school in the 1970s, my faculty department argued against my participation in their program, suggesting that I did not have what it took to be a mental health professional, although when asked, could not name any task or skill that I could not perform. This was a harsh lesson I experienced in being disrespected, which allowed me to resonate with the gang members who angrily spoke about being dissed. It directed my work toward a career of developing RFT. Many such minority groups, be they based on race, religion, nationality, gender, sexual orientation, or disability, have been and are still similarly minimalized.

We've all experienced disrespect at various times and ways throughout our lifetimes.

Disrespect is damaging whether it is in the form of discrimination, hatred, bullying, marginalization, rudeness, bias, neglect, or emotional, sexual or physical abuse. The only antidote, as I see it, is the infusion of healthy, grounded respect for all human beings.

Therapists have two important means of assisting clients achieve the more desirable outcome of feeling more respected and therefore being more capable of respecting others. Our first and most crucial aim, in this regard, is to attend to our respect for our clients with focused intention. This may seem to us to be assumed protocol, as we hopefully learned early in graduate school. We are told to be empathetic, non-biased, and supportive. I submit that to be focused on respect adds another layer, readdressing the meaning and purpose of the therapeutic relationship. There are subtle but clear differences between respect and empathy. To be empathetic is to be understanding of another's pain or anger or other emotions. This implies acceptance but doesn't directly offer recognition of another's values or core beliefs. Respect, however, does require that we check our own biases at the door and pay full attention to who this other person really is.

RFT is non-pathologic in approach. As a therapist, I am not looking for what's wrong with my client rather what is right and strong, that which can be built upon. My job is, above all, not only to establish a relationship that is indeed empathetic and supportive but also restorative and empowering, which necessarily includes providing the experience of being truly respected. I contend that this constitutes the majority of the healing process.

I say this with full recognition that there is more for us to do. We need to be aware of each client's goals, and help him or her achieve them using a full range of clinical skills, assessments, techniques, and so forth. In this process, though, the focus on respect can be woven into the dialog and experientially learned. If we keep in focus the underlying theme of respect as we move through all of the other processes and stages of therapy, we will deepen and strengthen a sustainable outcome.

Works of many will be noted in this book, but two bodies of work are the primary underpinnings of what I'm offering here. Martin Buber's *I and Thou* and the classic work of psychotherapist Carl Rogers provide the roots and foundation for my current work for our profession. Here I add to that foundation the more recent research supporting my approach, wisdom coming from other previous clinicians and researchers, as well as my 40 years of experience as a practicing clinician might have to contribute.

Dr. Sara Lawrence Lightfoot, sociologist and professor of education, wrote a book in 2000, entitled *Respect,* in which she relates beautiful narrative stories about herself and other people she knows, revealing true respect in everyday action. The resonating theme throughout is that respect "creates symmetry." Symmetry, as I conceptualize it, is about balance, unity, and genuine harmony. These words may seem like fantasy to many. I challenge that skepticism by offering that we can work toward that goal through the lens of RFT and be pleasantly surprised by our successes.

This book unfolds in the following way:

Chapter 1 is an introduction to the meaning and purpose of RFT, including the definition of respect as it is used in this context. It describes the subtle but significant differences between respect and empathy. The importance of the therapeutic relationship is emphasized, showing the dangers in power inequity of helping behavior.

Chapter 2 carries the importance of therapeutic relationship into the process of therapy. Introducing the subject of respect in a slow, gentle way through nondirective communication is fundamental to this transition. Applications of RFT in individual, couples, family, group therapy, transpersonal or universal respect, and social justice are introduced.

Chapter 3 focuses on honoring the pain that is brought into the room. Grief and trauma are the primary causes of the pain, and the resulting emotional injury, posttraumatic stress disorder (PTSD), often results from aggressive acts such as bullying or violence. Various means of therapeutic intervention, such as emotion-focused therapy (EFT), eye movement desensitization reprocessing (EMDR), and cognitive-behavior therapy (CBT), are considered from the RFT perspective.

Chapter 4 discusses healing the pain through rebuilding personal respect. Respect is carefully distinguished from esteem, which is subjectively self-reported, externally based, and temporal. Respect, in contrast, is grounded in core beliefs, dignity, integrity, meaning, and purpose.

Chapter 5 explains the complexity of doing couples work, which addresses the needs of the relationship as well as the needs of each individual. The interconnections among respect, trust, and intimacy are explored.

Chapter 6 describes the RFT approach to doing family therapy, introducing the complexity in working with families, due to the numerous combinations of relationships, which can co-occur within the family system as well as the entire system dynamics.

Chapter 7 offers ways in which RFT is useful in group process and cohesion. Four of Yalom's factors for group process—hope, universality, altruism, and interpersonal learning—are aligned with the tenets of RFT.

Chapter 8 addresses the larger picture: transpersonal, or universal, respect. Multiculturalism, the understanding of a wide variety of cultural differences, is held as an ethics issue by the code of ethics of all mental health professional associations. The areas of cultural differences discussed are race, ethnicity and nationality, religion and spirituality, gender and gender identity, disabilities, ageism, and poverty.

Chapter 9 addresses the necessity of self-care by therapists. An ethical issue addressed by all mental health codes of ethics, this is critical because distress or fatigue can lead to burnout then impairment as a clinician. Self-care is discussed in three different ways: taking care of one's physical, psychological, and spiritual needs.

The conclusion is a summary of the main tenets in the body of this book, including the meaning and significance of respect to the field of psychotherapy. RFT is also presented in summary, what it is, and how it can enhance the successes in our work.

Acknowledgments

I am deeply grateful to all the people who patiently supported me throughout this writing process. My first big thanks is to my lifetime friend, teacher, and mentor, Steen Halling at Seattle University, who has graciously given me many hours of his scholarly critique and support throughout this entire project.

My huge gratitude also goes to Richard Hoag for helping me design diagrams and reading several chapters—likewise to all who took the time to review various chapters: Lori Rowlett, Norma Leban, Susan Ducloux, Megan Van Meter, Stephen McCown, Sallie Ingle, Alexxe De Marco, Kali Gossett, Teana Harrington, Samantha Bond, Elizabeth Williams, and Frances Shelby. My thanks also goes to John V. Jones at St. Edwards University, Gena Minnix at Seminary of the Southwest, and Diane Harvey for reviewing my proposal, which opened the door for me to go on this marvelous journey.

Finally, thanks to my husband, Redge, who has endured these many months of book writing; my father, Cooper, for his encouragement; and my dearest friend, David, who also has stuck with me throughout.

1 Setting the Stage

The "I-Thou" Therapeutic Relationship

Respect is basic and essential to any positive human interaction. We all need and seek it. And yet, respect seems often to be lacking in a deeply harmful way in our world, our homes, our workplaces, and our communities. This phenomenon is often overlooked in therapy. We, who are in the mental health field, need to take a harder, more deliberate look at how we can best facilitate our clients establish the awareness and skills necessary to get it back.

We find examples of the lack of respect in the everyday lives of many of our clients, such as apathy in communication and listening skills in many relationships, serious disregard for the feelings of others, meanness in speech, or violent communication, as well as violent actions and abuse. The connections among these various levels of disrespectful behavior often seem to be understudied and therefore not addressed fully. In this chapter, we focus on these connections and the patterns they create to better understand the powerful strength of intervention respect can have as well as the danger and malignancy disrespect, unrecognized and untreated, imposes.

Respect is not only a noun but is also, and more powerfully, an active verb, requiring an intentional action of some sort. It can be as small as making eye contact with a pleasant smile or greeting or not interrupting someone speaking—simply good manners or polite behavior, as many think it to be. But it can be so much more, exceeding form or cordiality, becoming as deep as being tolerant and accepting of others' behavior or understanding of varying human perspectives, such as sexual or cultural differences. Regardless, respect can serve as a healing agent, making every human interaction work more effectively.

Respect-Focused Therapy (RFT) is not a technique or a theoretical model but rather a foundation on which all modalities and techniques used in therapy are, or should be, grounded to produce sound, effective outcomes. For the remainder of this chapter, I will be considering other theoretical approaches as they relate to RFT, how they are supportive through similarities, as well as how RFT brings additional perspective, unifying all of these approaches through the lens of respect.

The Therapist in the Therapist-Client Relationship

What the therapist brings to the therapist-client relationship is vitally important to the entire process and outcome of therapy. Because of the power disparity between therapist and client, it is easy to slip into the position of judge or parent without intention. Even the smallest biases can get in the way of doing good, effective work, such as regarding physical appearance, dress, hygiene, or language, not to mention parenting or relating styles or what we may consider to be inappropriate behaviors.

Our role as therapists inherently contains a certain power that can be too easily forgotten. We are the helpers, the professionals. We have been trained to be empathetic. We have learned skills and techniques. More importantly, the truth is, or should be, that we really do care, or we probably would not have chosen this field. We genuinely want to help alleviate human pain and suffering. It is with this intention that we go forward with this challenging but rewarding work. But the best intentions can be maligned by the presumption that we are indeed fulfilling this appropriately. This presumption can and does often bypass the focus of respect. The act of helping can then unintentionally create imbalance in power or asymmetry.

To this point, respect can become the equalizer, or as Lawrence-Lightfoot (2000) put it, respect "creates symmetry" (p. 5). One of the core principles of respect I present in this book is that respect in its truest form is not hierarchical; it is lateral and genuine and thereby most effective in creating real change. It is freely given, not demanded or fear based. This directly challenges one of the more widely assumed aspects of respect: that it is reserved for elders or authority. This assumption leaves out a large section of humanity, namely, all of those who do not have power or authority over others, including children.

In undergraduate school, I was required to write a senior-year thesis in psychology. I chose to do a phenomenological study of the nature of helping behavior, particularly as it related to the level of acceptability of the way the help was presented to the persons being helped. The two groups I studied were persons with physical disabilities and persons without obvious disabilities. It was particularly interesting to me that the nondisabled population found it harder to accept help than the disabled population did but just as notable, and perhaps more significantly to the point being made here, is that the factor that made help most acceptable to both groups was the feeling of equality with the helper. Condescension of any form made the help less desirable to those being helped. Being treated or perceived as helpless or inferior in any way most often was the cause of refusal of help.

As therapists, as human beings in this role, we need to remind ourselves always of our humanity, our own frailties, woundedness, triggers, biases, and perceptions of the world at large. The respect we have, or don't have, for ourselves is critical to how we find and build respect for our clients. Self-care, then, is a mandatory piece of the puzzle in the quality of care that we give to our clients. Our physical and mental well-being contribute heavily to our ability to be fully present and separate in a way that gives us the maximum capacity to openly respect the total uniqueness of the person(s) sitting in front of us. If we genuinely have respect for our unique selves, we are much more available to have it for others. There will be a more indepth discussion about how to gain and maintain this kind of self-care and real respect for oneself in the last chapter of this book, but from this point forward, please keep in mind that you are key in the entire process and development of RFT.

Mindfulness and Respect

With this self-awareness, it is important to be consistently mindful that the positive aspect of helping is evident when it is acknowledged as truly being helpful in a way that is wanted and balanced. By really listening to our desired path and outcome in therapy, we increase our ability to actually help in a much more significant way.

In recent years, much has been written and researched regarding mindfulness in therapy, as studied through the lenses interpersonal neurobiology and neural integration (Siegal, 2010). Mindfulness is about being fully aware in the present, both of self and others. It also includes "being open minded and avoiding premature closure of possibilities" (Langer, as cited in Siegal, 2010, p. 20) as well as "being aware, on purpose and nonjudgmentally, of what is happening, as it is happening in the present moment" (p. 20). All three definitions complement the meaning of respect as presented in this work, although they stop short of addressing the valued totality of others as well as self.

Allan Schore (2012) states, "Relational-affective processes between patient and therapist are at the core of the change mechanism. Indeed, a large body of basic research in clinical psychology on the therapeutic alliance is supporting a shift from a purely intrapsychic one-person psychology to a relational two-person psychology" (p. 10). I would submit that the work of Carl Rogers, which precedes this work, researched and postulated similar findings and therefore is foundational to it.

Being aware of one's nervous system status and how this affects and is affected by others' nervous systems have been covered extensively by the likes of Allan Schore and Dan Siegel, yet very little has been written specifically on the topic of respect as a central agent of change at both nonconscious and conscious levels in the therapeutic process. The practice of mindfulness-based therapy and the practice of RFT share parallels within the brain and might at first seem hard to distinguish, but there are substantial differences. The primary operational difference between the two approaches is that respect takes the affective focus of mindfulness to a new level by providing a cognitive template that seeks to realize that which is positive in self and others. Although this search for the positive might at first seem like a hearkening to Seligman's positive psychology, RFT is inherently focused on relationships with self and others, whereas positive psychology tends to focus on frame of mind and thus is not generally regarded as being relationally oriented.

Respect Versus Empathy

The etymology of the word *respect* is *respectare* or *respicere* (Latin derivation), meaning "to look again." To take another look, to reconsider, is to respect. In other words, to respect is to respond in a way that can create affirmation rather than dissent. It requires us to be willing to stand back, take another look, and reconsider that which is around us as well as inside of us. This reconsideration involves both cognitive and emotional processing, which take in the entirety of person, not just the presenting portion that is in front of us. In doing this, we can more effectively connect and build value in ourselves, in others, and in our world.

Empathy is derived from the Greek *en patheos*, which means "in feeling." Therefore, empathy is about shared understanding of emotion. This is a critical component in any therapeutic environment, requiring both learned skill and an innate human quality in the therapist. Experience is probably the best teacher of empathic understanding because it is so based in emotive connection, requiring vulnerability. We know that empathy is one of the most highly researched components of psychotherapy, yet still it is debated in terms of being more or less significant in the healing process as compared to specific technique or modality (Patterson, 1984).

Respect, conversely, has been much less researched in our field, even though Marie Jahada, (1958) (as cited by Hymer, 1987) recognized it as being "one of the major criteria for mental health" (p. 6). Dr. Sharon Hymer, one of a few to directly address the role of respect in psychotherapy, went on to say, "There have only been a few investigations of how therapists foster or impede the development of respect in psychotherapy. Respect concerns how we look at our patients and takes into account their uniqueness" (p. 6). Respect can expand the therapist's understanding of the client's experiential knowledge based on previous life events.

Furthermore, according to Dr. Ana Maria Rizzuto (1993), "[R]espect is naturally presumed to be a component of the therapeutic relationship. Therapists, however, need to go beyond the everyday understanding of respect and be prepared to provide a dimension that we do not expect to find in other human relations" (p. 277). She emphasized that respect is "the act of noticing with attention" (p. 277).

Respect encompasses empathy, requiring it to exist, yet goes far beyond empathy because it includes cognitive as well as affective understanding. Respect is a comprehensive understanding of a complete individual, including values, beliefs, culture, life experience, and the understanding and interpretation of that experience. Empathy is essential in establishing a connection to be built on, but respect carries that connection deeper and wider. To be clear, respect without empathy would be hollow, mechanical, and academic at best so that both must exist to firmly establish trust as well as connection.

Feminist Psychology

The feminist movement in the 1960s and 1970s had a profound impact on the culture of male dominance and, more significantly, on the empowerment of women. Although it certainly did not eradicate sexism, it did shine a bright light on the darker qualities of unfairness and inequality between the sexes, which opens doors for reevaluation of gender roles and their values in our society. As the feminist movement grew, it found new ground in psychotherapy as therapists found a new voice and determined ways to bring this voice into their work and share it with their clients. This shift in gender role assessment also led the way toward an even larger paradigm shift, which became inclusive of a wider definition of power disparity.

Dr. Laura Brown (2014) summarizes the development in feminist therapy in this way:

> Feminist Therapy is a theory that derives its inspiration and its wisdom from an in-depth interrogation of standpoints that are unavailable to dominant cultural simply because they have been relegated to the margins; the standpoints of Euro American women, people of color, lesbian, gay, and bisexual people, gender variant people, poor people, people with disabilities, immigrants and refugees.

This radical stance of listening more to the marginalized, or weaker voice, was not initially well received by mainstream psychology and still is primarily practiced by feminists, although the tenets of inclusion have been more normalized over the decades.

However, Brown goes further by establishing the fact that feminist therapy is not only inclusive of the marginalized but "privileges" or centers focus on the nondominant voice of wisdom.

> Feminist therapy does not simply study the "other" in order to offer a neutral perspective on that experience. Rather, what is inherent in Feminist Therapy theory is the radical notion that silenced voices of marginalized people are considered to be the sources of the greatest wisdom.
>
> (Brown, 2014)

The very notion that the persons least recognized become instead most valued by the process indicates an intention to reassess human worth and dignity not based on social norms, as is noted biblically as "the last shall be first and the first last." Again, respect is utilized to "reconsider" that which might not be apparent in other circumstances. Yet this primary shift in perspective serves to clarify and enrich the very meaning of human experience.

Vulnerability and Shame

Dr. Brene Brown (2013) has recently done interesting research on vulnerability and shame. She defines vulnerability as "uncertainty, risk and emotional exposure" (p. 34). She further says,

> Vulnerability is also the cradle of the emotions and experiences that we crave. Vulnerability is the birthplace of love, belonging, joy, courage, empathy, and creativity. It is the source of hope, empathy, accountability, and authenticity. If we want greater clarity in our purpose or deeper and more meaningful spiritual lives, vulnerability is the path.
>
> (p. 34)

Therefore, as difficult and uncomfortable as vulnerability may be, to risk emotional exposure, it is ultimately strength in being human and being open to real feelings and greater connection. We are most honored by clients who allow us into their place of vulnerability, and in turn, we need to honor them back by fully acknowledging their courage and their pain.

Of course, the difficult thing about being vulnerable is the fear of being shamed for it or by it. When you put out your naked real self, you lose your defense cover, making yourself more susceptible to the possibility of being shamed, which many of our clients are already too familiar with. The experience of being shamed by others often leads to internal shame, which is what therapists predominantly are charged to assist in repairing.

About shame, Brown (2013) suggests the way to dismantle it: "If we cultivate enough awareness about shame to name it and speak to it, we've basically cut it off at the knees. Shame hates having words wrapped around it. If we speak shame, it begins to wither" (p. 58).

Thus, our job seems to be about honoring vulnerability while helping give voice to, name, and call out the shame for the purpose of depowering it, not adding to it. We may not like or accept everything our clients do or say, but it is our ethical responsibility to honor them as fellow human beings, not to shame them further. As unintentional as this may be, we need to be ever vigilant and more purposeful to avoid creating additional shame because of the blind trust and heightened vulnerability our clients bring to us in the therapeutic process. Consistently mindful of this built-in authority or power, we have to use it with wisdom and great care in this unusually fragile relationship.

Humanistic Existentialism

Mental health diagnoses can also get in our way of respecting the whole person because we may consider persons who have the more complex or challenging ones, such as bipolar disorder, chemical addiction, or borderline personality disorder, as being primarily defined by that diagnosis and to be more difficult or bothersome because of it. We, too, are human and subject to our own biases, but we need to keep a close check on them, as they may have subtle, or not so subtle, negative impacts on the therapeutic process.

Regarding this problem with mental health diagnoses, Yalom (2014) gives a very clear example:

> What? "Borderline patients play games?" That is what you said? Ernest, you'll never be a real therapist if you think like that. That's exactly what I meant earlier when I talked about the dangers of diagnosis. There are borderlines and there are borderlines. Labels do violence to people. You can't treat the label; you have to treat the person behind the label.
>
> (p. 17)

Humanistic existential therapy has its roots from the mid-20th century, most notably from the works of Yalom and May, and is based in great part on the works of Kierkegaard, philosopher and theologian from the 1800s.

Daniel Pitchford (2009) describes existential therapy this way:

> The purpose of existential therapy is to confront the anxieties of daily living and create meaning from and connectedness to lived experiences. . . . The personal responsibility of existential therapists is to understand their clients' anxieties and experiences and to guide them through their struggles.
>
> (p. 441)

May was influenced by Kierkegaard's discussions of "fear of nothingness" or death or lack of meaning and purpose. Hence, his focus in therapy was to "guide" clients toward their own meaning and truth. This meant that truth is individually subjective and should be understood in that context.

The concept of subjective meaning hits at the very heart of RFT. To not have preformulated truths, but to allow for other's truths to exist concurrently, yet separately from your own, is essential to fully respect, as we will see through the works of Buber and Rogers.

The "I-Thou" Relationship and Unconditional Regard

RFT is largely couched in the works of Martin Buber and Carl Rogers. Martin Buber, a Hasidic Jewish theologian and philosopher who wrote from the early 1900s and throughout the majority of that century, wrote a classic piece of literature called *I and Thou*. In this writing, Buber (1987) contrasts the "I-Thou" relationship with the "I-It" relationship. In describing the difference between "Thou" and "It," Buber said, " 'It' is bounded by others; 'it' exists only through being bounded by others. But when 'Thou' is spoken, there is nothing. 'Thou' has no bounds" (p. 4).

In looking at the complexity of relationships, Buber not only looks at to what or whom I relate but, more importantly, how I relate to the other person. If I treat another as an "It," an object of my need or perception, I put limitations on that individual, objectifying him or her rather than experiencing another human being. This objectification stems from one's own needs, wants, prejudices, or other agendas.

To be open to the Thou experience is much more risky in the sense that one relinquishes control in the relationship, allowing the other to be truly and completely other, separately whole, not in any way scripted by one's expectations. As rare an experience as Buber said this is, it is perhaps the most freeing to suspend all preconception and design to observe and absorb another's reality untainted by one's own.

To be sure, it takes emotional courage, energy, and strength to be able to make oneself so vulnerable, so candidly emotionally exposed to another's humanity. Therapists are real people who have real limits on this kind of courage and strength, but as much as humanly possible, we owe it to our clients and to ourselves to be truly present in the therapeutic relationship, permitting ourselves to be openly available to the I and the Thou in perhaps the most intensely critical, transforming interchange for our clients. Although the focus is always to be squarely on the well-being of the client, we can also be evolving forward in this process. It has been my experience that the more practiced I become in allowing myself to enter this kind of relationship, the more inviting and less daunting it becomes.

In this way, we can better model for parents how not to make their children objects of their own hopes or dreams, for partners how not to overlay their past familial experiences onto their current relationships, or for individuals how not to devalue themselves at their core by someone else's measures.

Nonrecognition of human value, as innocent as it may seem in the moment, as a pattern of behavior emerges, often has manipulative and damaging effects, such as relating to others as sex objects, as objects for economic gain, or simply as objects for power or control.

Working with manipulators and abusers is very challenging work, at least for me. To stretch my I-Thou capacity to encompass persons whom I know or experience as being systematically abusive, either passive aggressively or aggressively, I internally squirm at the notion of maintaining any sense of Thou with this person who has no idea what Thou is anyway and doesn't seem to care.

But relating to the Thou is not conditional. Buber said, "Thou have no bounds" (Buber, Martin, & Smith, 1987, p. 4). As difficult as it may be, my application of this same approach needs to be consistent. As long as I also maintain and nurture the "I" that is in me, to be healthy and strong, the possibility of being harmed emotionally is minimized. Respecting self as well as other is essential in this entire process. When I am able to keep a solid balance of self and other, permitting my safety while continuing to honor the other, I have a much greater chance at unlocking the real Thou in that other person, not only through my eyes but also through that person's understanding as well.

Adame & Leitner (2009) wrote about "reverence" in therapy in a similar manner as I am presenting the concept of respect. They explained experiential personal construct psychotherapy (EPCP) in the following manner: "According to EPCP, one of the highest levels of psychological functioning is the ability to revere another person in a relationship, and the experience of connecting with someone on such an intimate level is healing in and of itself" (p. 253).

This underscores the strikingly essential effect of reverence or respect. I see these two words in a parallel way. Although they do not have the exact same meanings, they seem to carry at least similar intent. Reverence has, perhaps, a stronger tone, carrying with it a more spiritual connotation. Respect, though, as I see it, has the same potency of meaning with or without spiritual overtones and has more teachable constructs for mutuality in everyday practice. Regardless, the points made by this model seem to strengthen the positions of RFT as well.

In almost a poetic, very beautiful way, EPCP describes the role of the therapist from the client perspective: Leitner (as cited in Adame & Leitner, 2009) explains, "[R]everence implies awareness that the other is 'holding my heart respectfully, treating my soul gently, and seeing the decency behind my shame and my retreats from others' " (p. 255). In turn, he describes that same interaction from the therapist's perspective: "We also recognize the profound gift the other person is giving us by trusting us with his or her most central aspects of being, knowing that by doing so we have the choice of either validating or invalidating those essential constructs of ourselves" (p. 255).

They build on this notion of gaining a sense of worthiness in the therapeutic relationship by explaining how the client can become his or her own "active meaning-maker":

> In this I-Thou stance, a person is open to the world and engages it as an active meaning-maker. . . . Thus, within the therapy relationship the client may become more experientially aware of an array of constructive alternatives previously unknown to him or her.
>
> (p. 256)

We might have to look a little harder to recall examples of the I-Thou experiences in our own lives, but we have them. When I look into the eyes of my nieces and nephews, I frequently experience the I-Thou with them because their love is so simple and basic. We just need to be there to enjoy each other. People who are in love, with any luck, will experience the Thou with their mates at least a handful of times, if not many more, during their journeys together. People who experience God usually report having an I-Thou kind of spiritual experience.

Because I-Thou may imply intimacy, it is our job as therapists to create the environment and the opportunity for just this level of relating to occur, within professional boundaries—no romantic overtones permitted, of course. Furthermore, we need to be willing to open ourselves to this process and initiate the kind of interaction that comfortably invites the client to participate and maybe experience for the first time, or at least at a crucial time, the empowerment of being treated as a Thou rather than an It. If we look for the Thou in others, we are more likely to find it, but it takes trained intentional focus. It also demands of us, as professionals, a certain level of emotional energy and vulnerability, which we typically do not extend beyond our loved ones.

Balancing this kind of emotional extension to our clients with good, healthy boundaries, which maintain the therapeutic value of this unique relationship, is paramount. We must be careful to avoid any duality in this relationship, that is, friendship on any social level, romance, or a business relationship. As artificial or awkward as this might appear to be at first glance, this very structured framework, when based in genuine sincerity, allows for growth and progress for the client and sometimes for the therapist as well.

If respect means to look again, perhaps it also means the removal of preconceptions, expectations, judgments, or needs, replacing them with a continual willingness to reevaluate or reconsider our assumptions. Perhaps it means allowing for the I-Thou experiences to be uniquely separate and the meaning and value of each to deepen in the relationship.

The I-Thou relationship, then, lends itself to the notion of what many call love. In *The Four Loves,* C. S. Lewis (1960), a prolific Christian writer, reinforces these concepts by describing several different kinds of love, including what he calls "Gift Love" and "Need Love." About the contrast of these two kinds of love, Lewis says, "The typical example of Gift Love would be that love which moves a man to work and save for the future well-being of his family which he will die without sharing or seeing; of the second, that which sends a lonely or frightened child into the arms of his mother!" (p. 63). Gift Love, then, is what therapists have to offer—that love which does not expect any return but is offered only as a conduit for positive change.

Respect can only grow out of nurturing positive regard for self and others. Carl Rogers, a well-known psychotherapist in the 1960s and 1970s, in his most popular book, *On Becoming a Person* (1991), describes his sense of respect, "unconditional positive regard," as "a caring, which is not possessive. It demands all persons, with permission, to have their own feelings and experiences, and to find their own meaning to it" (p. 283).

Rogers (1991) articulates beautifully and precisely the very essence of the respect I seek to have with every client:

> I find that the more acceptance and liking I feel toward this individual, the more I will be creating a relationship which he can use. By acceptance I mean a warm regard for him as a person of unconditional self-worth—of value no matter what his condition, his behavior, or his feelings. It means a respect and liking for him as a separate person, a willingness for him to possess his own feelings in his own way. It means an acceptance of and regard for his attitudes of the moment, no matter how negative or positive, no matter how much they may contradict other attitudes he has held in the past. This acceptance of each fluctuating aspect of this other person makes it for him a relationship of warmth and safety, and the safety of being liked and prized as a person seems a highly important element in a helping relationship.
>
> (p. 34)

To work with unconditional positive regard means accepting our differences, whatever they might be—race, gender, sexual orientation, disability, religion, nationality, or any other kind of arbitrary exclusion of others from the opportunity for being experienced positively. This, in fact, is what is known as cultural competency or diversity, which is hugely relevant in today's world, in all health care, education, business, society, politics, or international affairs. As with other professionals, therapists have an obligation to maintain the highest ethic in this arena of competency.

Think about what kind of world we might be able to live in if more teachers could have this kind of regard for their students, parents could share it with each of their children, and civic and religious leaders could model it for the groups they represent. We, as therapists, have a unique opportunity to pass forward respectful behavioral and attitudinal perceptual changes by implementing them in this delicate process called therapy.

Fortunately, there are emerging models currently that are echoing many of these concerns and needs. In education, there is a relatively new model in academic planning called the Person Centered Plan (Holburn & Vietze, 2002). In the medical field (Ekman et al., 2011), hospitals and nursing homes are starting to consider patient—or person—centered care, which focuses on the goals of each individual patient in their care rather than predetermined, standardized protocols based on diagnoses, set by medical staff. In the legal profession, there is a new program called restorative justice (Zehr, 2015), which speaks to the needs of victims of crimes by addressing specifically the relationship between victim and perpetrator using social work and therapeutic interventions. Finally, from within the field of mental health, there are innovative movements like recovery mental health and Heart and Soul of Change Project.

Person-Centered Planning and Care

Similar to and fashioned after Roger's client-centered approach is a more current trend of person-centered planning and care (Adams & Grieder, 2004), which stretches beyond the field of mental health into education as well as broader health care services. The concept is relatively simple: that the "patient" or "client" or "student" is indeed a person and ought to be fully regarded as such, thereby as fully included in treatment or education planning and goal setting as possible. As straightforward as this may appear, it is indeed a paradigm shift, particularly as it relates to the medical model because that model is premised in the idea that the doctor is the expert and the patient is to follow the doctor's orders.

From within the mental health arena, the shift in power and responsibility from being strictly on the side of the service provider to being shared in partnership with the patient or consumer suggests that not only is this model more desirable for the client's self-regard; it is actually more effective in creating better outcomes (Zehr, 2015).

Recovery Mental Health

Recovery mental health incorporates and builds on person-centered planning and care by asserting that the recovery model as used in addiction treatment can be used effectively also with the chronically mentally ill. Again, research is being done by the aforementioned institutions with favorable results.

As cited by Larry Davidson (2014), Phillippe Pinel began the concept of recovery of mental illness in 1794 by saying in a presentation:

> One cannot ignore a striking analogy in nature's ways when one compares the attacks of intermittent insanity with the violent symptoms of an acute illness. It, in either case, would be a mistake to measure the gravity, to measure the danger, by the extent of the trouble and derangement of the vital functions. In both cases a serious condition may forecast recovery, provided that one practices prudent management.
>
> (p. 729)

Pinel went on to say that "to consider madness as a usually incurable illness is to assert a vague proposition that is constantly refuted by the most authentic facts." And yet those preconceptions, "errors," and "prejudices," according to Pinel, the incomprehensibility of the mentally ill, the total pervasiveness, and the incurability of the illness are still perpetuated today in the traditional medical model (Davidson, Rakfeldt, and Strauss, 2011).

However, recovery is having a resurgence in research and practice. Patricia Deegan (2014), psychologist and advocate of the recovery movement, refers to recovery as the "Conspiracy of Hope" because it empowers the person living with mental illness to partner and participate in his or her own treatment. She talks about "personal medicine" as being the steps of self-care, like listening to music to drown out the voices or taking walks to soothe anxiety, that is, having a voice in the entire treatment plan. Recovery is strength based, socially just, and holistic and provides moral treatment. This model utilizes peer specialists who have lived experiences with mental illness but who are also trained to support and advocate for the person in treatment. This helps equalize the power in the therapeutic relationship and creates more room for self-determination for the client.

It is important to point out that whereas this model is initially set to assist those with more critical mental illnesses, like schizophrenia and bipolar disorder, it can be well utilized by any population because at its base, recovery is about the civil rights of the client and, ultimately, self-determination. To this end, it underscores and validates RFT. Respect for the client as a whole person with strengths and assets as well as weakness can indeed help them be more empowered to take responsibilities for improving their own lives.

An offshoot of the recovery model is the Heart and Soul of Change Project. Its primary objective is to determine what is perceived as being beneficial in an individual's therapy, according to that person, the client, or the participant, as this model refers to them.

Dr. Barry Duncan, founder of this approach, has written several books and articles relating to and explaining its rationale. In his newest book, *On Becoming a Better Therapist* (2014), he begins by describing the importance of the therapeutic relationship thusly:

> I have been privileged to witness the irrepressible ability of human beings to transcend adversity—clients troubled by self-loathing and depression, battling alcohol or drugs, struggling with intolerable marriages, terrorized by inexplicable voices, oppressed by their children's problems, traumatized by past or current life circumstances, and tormented with unwanted thoughts and anxieties—with amazing regularity. . . . Regardless of discipline, theoretical persuasion, or career level, they really care about people and strive to do good work. The odds for change when you combine a resourceful client and caring therapist are worth betting on, certainly cause for hope, and responsible for my unswerving faith in psychotherapy as a healing endeavor.
>
> (p. 5)

However, Duncan points out starkly that we have few real markers for improvement in our work including those we most often rely on: trainings and continuing education in the latest trends in techniques or modalities, personal therapy, or even our experience as clinicians, citing research from a number of clinicians.

What Duncan points to as being the best indicator of true improvement is the direct feedback from clients about their own perceptions of their benefit from therapy. He has developed an outcome rating scale, which clients fill out after each session, stating how effective they feel that session was in their therapy. Whether one takes to this kind of rating system or not, the point for therapists to grasp is to rely on our clients for the best source of outcome feedback. This reflects the very intention of RFT.

RFT, as the presented research indicates, is well supported by previous and contemporary scholars in this field. So far we have examined the therapeutic relationship as it is the most critical underpinning of this approach. But this is not the totality of what RFT offers. It needs to go beyond the relationship into the heart of the process of therapy to maximize the potential for real and lasting change for our clients.

RFT offers something substantially different, beyond much of the previously mentioned research. For the remainder of this book, we will explore the ways in which the therapeutic process can significantly progress as the central theme of respect is brought into the room. The therapeutic relationship lays the foundation of respect but necessarily leads that experience of being respected toward healing and the awareness of the positive power of respect in everyday life.

References

Adame, Alexandra L., & Leitner, Larry M. (2009). Reverence and recovery: Experiential personal construct psychotherapy and transpersonal reverence. *Journal of Psychology, 22*, 253–257.

Adams, N., & Grieder, D. M. (2004). *Treatment planning for person-centered care: The road to mental health and addiction recovery*. Salt Lake City, UT: Academic Press.

Brown, Brene. (2013). *Daring greatly: How the courage to be vulnerable transforms the way we live, love, parent, and lead*. New York: Penguin.

Brown, L. (2014, October 20). Feminist therapy. Retrieved from www.laurabrown.com

Buber, Martin, & Smith, R. G. (translator). (1987). *I and Thou*. New York: Scribner-Macmillan.

Davidson, L., Rakfeldt, J., & Strauss, J. (2011). *The roots of the recovery movement in psychiatry: Lessons learned*. New York: John Wiley & Sons.

Davidson, L. What You need to Know About Evidence Base for Mental Health Recovery. Presented to the Hogg Foundation for Mental Health Robert Lee Sutherland Seminar XVIII, Austin, TX 2014.

Deegan, P. Personal Medicine, Power Statements and Other Disruptive Innovations. Presented to the Hogg Foundation for Mental Health Robert Lee Sutherland Seminar XVIII, Austin, TX 2014.

Duncan, B. L. (2014). *On becoming a better therapist, second edition: Evidence-based practice one client at a time*. New York: American Psychological Association.

Ekman, I., Swedberg, K., Taft, C., Lindseth, A., Norberg, A., Brink, E., . . . & Lidén, E. (2011). Person-centered care—Ready for prime time. *European Journal of Cardiovascular Nursing, 10*(4), 248–251.

Holburn, S., & Vietze, P. (Eds.). (2002). *Person-centered planning: Research, practice, and future directions*. Baltimore, MD: Paul H Brookes Publishing Company.

Hymer, S. (1987). Respect in psychotherapy. *Journal of Contemporary Psychotherapy, 17*(1), 6–15.

Jahoda, M. (1958). *Current concepts of positive mental health*. New York: Basic Books.

Lawrence-Lightfoot, S. (2000). *Respect*. New York: Perseus Books.

Lewis, C. S. (1960). *The four loves*. New York: Harcourt, Brace.

Patterson, C. H. (1984). Empathy, warmth, genuineness, in psychotherapy: A review of reviews. *Psychotherapy, 21*(4), 431–438.

Pinel, P. Memoir into Madness: A Contribution to the Natural History of Man. Presented to the Society for Natural History, Paris, France 1794.

Pitchford, D. B. (2009). The existentialism of Rollo May. *Journal of Humanistic Psychology, 49*(4), 441–461.

Rizzuto, A. (1993). Respect in clinical practice. *Journal of Psychotherapy Practice and Research*, 2: 4, 277–279.

Rogers, C. R. (1991). *On becoming a person: A therapist's view of psychotherapy*. New York: Houghton Mifflin Co.

Schore, A. N. (2012). *The science of the art of psychotherapy*. New York: W. W. Norton & Company.

Siegal, D. J. (2010). *The mindful therapist*. New York: W. W. Norton & Company.

Yalom, I. D. (2014). *Lying on the couch: A novel*. New York: Basic Books.

Zehr, H. (2015). *The little book of restorative justice: Revised and updated*. New York: Skyhorse Publishing, Inc.

2 Establishing the Central Theme in the Process
Bringing Respect Into the Room

Carl Rogers stressed the therapeutic relationship as the primary agent for a healing process to occur. From the RFT perspective, this relationship must be present with intentional respect coming from the therapist. However, RFT also posits that it is equally important also to move the topic of respect into the heart of the therapeutic process and discussion as a primary theme. This should be done gently so as not to lose the established experience of a newly developed bond of respect with the client. To interject the subject of respect too quickly or forcefully may be received negatively—ironically, as being judgmental, dogmatic, or authoritative in manner. More appropriate to the dialog might be an interwoven thread of respect-focused questions, metaphors, storytelling, and so forth, which may elicit thoughts and feelings about being respected or disrespected or possibly about being respectful or disrespectful toward others. It is in the weaving of the discussion of respect into the particular issues and concerns presented by the client that we must pay extra attention to how we proceed.

Introducing Respect

The assumption made in the RFT approach is that the human brokenness, which is brought into the room, has its roots in the experience of profound disrespect in some or many ways. The healing of that brokenness comes in establishing, or reestablishing, an experiential, explicit comprehension of what respect really is and how it can be meaningful in the client's life going forward.

Respect develops over time, not all at once. My experience as a clinician has been that the concept of being respected, feeling respectable to oneself, or being able to respect others, has been significantly diminished in a typical client's life experience, such that when it is experienced in my office, it is fragile, and I need to treat carefully. If I neglect that sense of fragility, I risk clouding, if not overshadowing, the client's own thoughts and feelings about what's happening in the moment.

Introducing the first thread of the meaning of respect into the therapeutic process usually happens while gathering the story of what brought the client into your office in the first place. Typically, within the first session or two, a great deal of information is gathered, which can be initially used to assess the degree of respect or disrespect the client is experiencing or has experienced over a lifetime. In a simple summary, this understanding can be conveyed in a way as to be validating that the client's emotional pain through disrespect—abandonment, neglect, abuse, and so on—is clearly heard. This might be the first time the client has ever received that validation in a meaningful way. If this connection is made, then the foundation for gaining a deeper sense of respect is created. Bringing the client's attention to this may not require saying anything out loud. Doing so might seem to imply judgment to some clients who are particularly sensitive to the entire subject of respect. Rather, to acknowledge and support the client's new awareness nonverbally may be a stronger means of communication at this point.

Case in Point

I had seen Sheila three or four times. She was an African American woman in her late 30s, single with three kids, and very chronically depressed with a history of childhood abandonment and abuse as well as having similar experiences with the men in her life. What brought her into my office was a Child Protective Services (CPS) report mandating counseling before she would be able to get her children back. She had begun to repeat the patterns she had learned as a child, leaving them for hours at time and hitting one with a hairbrush.

She was in a rush to get "this counseling mess over with," to get her kids back, although I had a sense she was connecting with me more than she would admit. She presented with a great deal of both anger and detachment, even when talking about her kids, although she repeated that she loved them very much in a flat affect presentation.

It was at this point that I made my first attempt to bring up respect in our conversation. I asked her what she most respected about her kids. She had little to say other than to more vigorously repeat how much she loved them. I then asked what she respected most about herself as a parent with her children. With this, I almost lost her. She blew up, saying that I was just like the rest of them (therapists). I didn't know how hard it was. She ran out of my office, was gone for 10 to 15 minutes, then came back, and remained silent for another 10 minutes or so. Finally, when she spoke, quietly she told me what a bad mother she was, what a bad person she was, just like her mother, and she wept profusely. I suggested that there might be another way to assess the situation, that is, that she may just lack the knowledge and skills that she never learned from her mother, which she needed to fulfill her concept of what a good mother should be. But she was not able to process this idea at this time and shut down. Soon after, we ended the session.

Fortunately, she came back the next week, telling me that she had thought about what I had said and that she thought that I could be right. We proceeded to work on parenting skills as well as her sense of self-respect. I had created a workable intervention, simply switching the problem from her perceived bad character to her need and desire to learn more effective parenting skills. This broke her defensive denial system but also encouraged her to find room for respect that she had never felt before. Had I continued to push her into believing that she was a good mother, at that moment, was so threatening for her to accept, I'm certain she would have discontinued therapy. The very idea that she had any worth, as a parent or otherwise, had been stripped away from her so severely by CPS, on top of her lack of receiving positive parenting as a child, that now to believe in herself as a parent was too frightening. Moving forward with her meant building confidence through much reinforcement while carefully placing suggestions for improvements where and when she could clearly receive them positively.

Reinforcement for the client's willingness to consider the construct of respect in any new regard needs to be gentle, incremental at first, allowing the client to process and notice it on his or her own terms. This often is slow to occur both because of the lack of familiarity with it for the client and the newness of the therapeutic relationship.

Understanding the Pain of Grief, Loss, and Trauma

Grief is complex and, as uniquely personal as it is, also universal. Each person responds to it in his or her own way, but we know, as Kubler-Ross (1969) clearly points out, that most grieving processes include denial, anger, bargaining, depression, and eventually some level of acceptance. We also know that so many variables affect this process: the nature and intensity of the loss or losses as well as the temperament, personality, and coping skills of the bereaved and the level of support available. And because grief so broadly covers such a wide array of losses, from death of a parent, spouse, child, or friend to divorce or other type of loss, such as a move, unemployment, illness, or a disability, it's difficult to pinpoint direction in therapy, except to stay with the client as he or she journeys through it. It is tempting to suggest that the client moves forward past where we feel stuck with him or her, past the denial, anger, or depression, but in doing so, we're robbing the client of his or her own healing process.

Case in Point

Mary, a 53-year-old African American woman, had lost her 17-year-old son, Johnny, first to drugs and then to police brutality, which led to his suicide. I had been his therapist on an inpatient basis for substance abuse. After several inpatient treatments, he was maintaining sobriety and starting to get his life back together, but he still had bouts of uncontrollable anger.

I had done some family work with Johnny and his mother in an inpatient treatment facility 6 months before his death. I learned at that time that Joshua's father had been an addict and had abandoned them when Joshua was four. His mother had struggled to make enough money to feed them both, but she continued to push him to do well in school and get a good education. Joshua struggled equally in school. It was later discovered that he had a learning disability, but the school did not provide the support he or his mother needed to understand or work with this problem. Other kids and some of the teachers bullied Joshua. He developed great frustration and depression to the point that he eventually dropped out of school and eventually began his drug addiction. During his third hospitalization, he was also diagnosed with bipolar disorder. Soon after this last discharge, he was walking home from his job when a police officer pulled up behind him in his car, turned on his siren, and ran into Joshua and one of his friends. The friend was killed instantly, and Joshua was in intensive care for weeks. A month or so later Joshua was in so much physical and emotional pain that he shot himself. He died hours later.

So after his death, she became my client. It was very evident to me that this was going to be extensive, long-term therapy because of the complex grief of losing a child to the kind of brutality Joshua had experienced before his death as well as in the way he died. I was also quite aware that it was going to be very intense because of the social injustice he and his mother, as well as his community, had received. I intentionally stayed quiet and just listened to her excruciating pain and lashing anger for months, growing into a year. The most difficult part for me was hearing her repeat, over and over again, every single detail of the death scene, which tragically, she had witnessed—the position of his body, the blood and brain particles all over the walls, and how all of that merged into the ongoing yet fresh burn created by such cruelty. This hateful and senseless act took place years before the Black Lives Matter movement occurred, but it was my introduction to the overwhelming realization that this is systemically the daily reality for far too many people.

> *Finally, after about 6 months, I started to suggest gently that maybe it was time to let that vision of the death scene fade and to focus on more positive memories of him with full recognition that the pain of her loss and the weight of the injustice would never really go away. She agreed that that was what she should do and earnestly tried with great difficulty.*
>
> *I continued working with her several more months, frequently validating that her memory of him and the circumstances that led up to that terrible day would always be significant for her. Her life had been forever robbed, preventing her from fully processing what had so dramatically changed her world.*

Grief and trauma often overlap; indeed, they frequently seem the same. Both are jarring and alter our realities forever forward, however we may be able to process them. Some grief events seem less traumatic than others, and some traumas appear to have little to do with grief, such as loss of a job, a chronic illness, or even observations of horrific events.

Nonetheless, both impact human existences in ways we never completely recover from or understand. We're learning more about the neuroscience of how the brain receives such injuries, and in fact, there are physical changes in the brain that we are now identifying as a part of posttraumatic stress disorder (PTSD), which will be discussed in more depth in the next chapter.

Rebuilding Self-Respect

Rebuilding self-respect is actually at the core of most individual therapy. It is frequently identified as a primary goal and yet often one of the most complex to attain. One's sense of self is often damaged through trauma, loss, or being repeatedly discounted and negated by others. Often, a client has moved from one wounding event to the next, not recovered from the last, and becomes retriggered and reinjured over and over again, compounding the level of damage done. This creates a tangled web of pain that becomes indefinable. Working through and sorting out that web is the goal in therapy.

It is one thing to address a singular painful event in one's life, such as a divorce, a death in the family, or loss of a job; however, those events usually are not so singular but contain clusters of other related events. When those events begin to domino and, in fact, dominate this person's existence, the pattern can begin to build into a belief system of pessimism and hopelessness. It is like a simple cold that turns into pneumonia with infectious complications. But this is not an illness; it is a human response to much suffering and may well become a lifelong pattern of misery without positive, respectful intervention.

In these cases, we can only hope to enter the client's reality and introduce the experience of respect to allow the client the opportunity to internalize the value of such and to begin incorporating it into his or her way of thinking about self and others. Mindful that our own expectations around such internalization may not be met in the way we might conceptualize, we can encourage and support any awareness or shift in the direction the client can comfortably find helpful. Keep in mind that this downward spiral of negative thinking has likely taken years to develop and will often be slow and difficult to reverse. We may never see the full fruits of the hoped for outcome, but we can watch as the seeds of change are planted.

However, it is indeed possible to intervene in this spiral, with respect. This intervention takes much patience, giving the client reinforcement of worthiness and value, as she or he is able to assimilate. It means sitting with the client and carefully supporting him or her in rediscovering, or discovering for the first time, those inner qualities and strengths that are presently unavailable. It further means to be able to help begin the integration of respect into one's self-identity as a part of a larger humanity—to understand that everyone deserves to have a sense of dignity regardless of who the person is or what he or she has done in the past.

The ability to genuinely find favor with oneself often, if not always, requires some sort of self-forgiveness for being human and having shortcomings. This alone frequently is difficult and can become a large part of the work. Beyond forgiveness is acceptance of one's imperfections and ownership of one's strengths and abilities. Regardless of methodology, Rogerian, CBT, EFT, and/or any other specific orientation, breaking through this self-inflicting yet tender barrier must be highly focused on respecting the whole person, including the brokenness.

Case in Point

Kelly, a 34-year-old Hispanic woman, came into therapy because she said, "I have disgraced my family. I have become a monster!" During the initial interview, it was difficult to get any specific details about how she had earned her claims to either be a disgrace to the family or a monster, but that did not dampen her certainty of the stated facts one bit. It was true, and that was that!

Tears, sobs, and yells of declaration of her insufficiencies as a person were uninterrupted for most of the session. I simply nodded and confirmed her pain. Toward the end of the session, I said, "You know, it takes a great deal of courage to face our shortcomings. We all have them, of course, but many of us are afraid to admit them. You strike me as a very brave woman!"

She stared at me in shock. Had I not heard her just tell me how horrible she was? I let her know that I heard how bad she thought she was, but however negative her actions were, whatever difficult circumstances she found herself in as a result, those things did not make her a bad person. Her face brightened into a small grin, and she thanked me.

I didn't see her again. A few months later, she called me to tell me that her husband had berated her for years, telling her what a bad wife, mother, housekeeper, and lover she was. Right before she came to see me, she had found evidence of another woman who had been in her house and had confronted her husband about it. He exploded on her, telling her that it was all her fault because she failed at being a woman and was no more than a dog. She had had enough and was finally leaving him.

On her way home from our appointment, she was so astonished that someone actually thought she was brave. She started thinking about her life married to this very mean man and realized how brave she actually was. She talked to her sister, who agreed, and said that she had been praying for her to recognize how cruel he had been all these years. Her sister helped her get a lawyer, move to her sister's city, and get a job far away from him. She knew then how brave she really could be.

Respect and Couples

Working with couples obviously creates more complexity to the task of doing therapy, simply by virtue of the fact that there is now more than one person in the room, each person having his or her unique life stories and needs, plus the relationship issues brought forward by them collectively. In 40 years of doing therapy, it becomes clearer to me that the primary goal in couples' therapy is almost always about addressing the lack of respect in some fashion or another, regardless of the presenting issues: infidelity, addiction, estrangement, verbal and/or physical abuse, or simply lack of communication skills—at least one person, usually both, feels disrespected in the relationship.

Sometimes working with couples is like juggling balls. Maintaining a balance of perspectives can be tricky as the therapist needs to pay full attention to each person as well as to the dynamics between them. When you can safely bring the theme of respect into the room such that the clients can each relate to it and use it effectively and fairly, the task becomes better directed.

Realizing that each person in the room has not only the present relationship to be worked out, but also a series of past relationships, including familial, which contribute to the present dynamics, again compounds the complexity of the work required. Helping the couple understand the connections of past and present, which weigh on their current situation, is significant (Hendrix, 2007). To do it in a way that is neither blaming nor shaming requires due diligence, both in terms of maintaining nonjudgment from the therapist perspective as well as guiding the dialog in such a way that awareness of nonviolent communication by each person is achieved. In other words, we are setting the stage for a new relational paradigm. This paradigm might, and often does, involve a new way of conversing through vocabulary, tone, and nonverbal interaction, which may not permit nonviolent communication to take a dominant place in the relationship.

Case in Point

Ron and Carol, both Caucasians in their 40s, came into therapy because "there is no trust left in their marriage," although they both say that they still love one another and want to save the marriage.

There is history of cheating on both sides and some reference to alcohol and drug abuse in the past. They have two children, a 14-year-old boy and a 12-year-old girl. They have both been married before.

Within 15 minutes, they are yelling and cursing at one another. The noise level is increasing by the second. I have an urge to blow a loud whistle like a referee would do, but instead I attempt to de-escalate the situation by softly suggesting a time-out. It takes a few minutes for them to hear me and respond, but eventually they settle, with a quizzical look at me. I ask each of them to summarize what the other one just said. They give a faulty attempt at following my request but fall back into their pattern of accusatory, violent communication quickly. I suggested that they think about the ways in which each of their parents communicated and whether or not they noticed any similar patterns in the way they were currently communicating. They both, rather embarrassed by this new realization, nodded yes.

It took more sessions, but they were slowly able to listen more to one another and integrate nonviolent verbal and body language into their conversations. The volume reduced significantly as well. It was only when they could and did intentionally listen to one another that the content in the dialogue shifted from blame to problem solving. The new sense of being respected gave each more safety in tackling the larger challenges in their relationship.

Respect in Family Systems

When working with families, the dimensions of necessary respect grow exponentially. Not only do we as therapists need to have the ability to respect each individual in the room, but we also need to understand and respect each of the dyads and triads that are playing out among all persons involved (Bowen, 1993). For example, if you have a family of four, Mom, Dad, Sister, and Brother, you then have the relationships between parents, siblings, Mom and Brother, Mom and Sister, Dad and Brother, and Dad and Sister as well as all the triads that can be made out of the four. So not only recognizing and tracking all of these relationships but also finding ways to truly honor each segment of the family, as well as the total dynamic presented as the family, is vital to the process. As complex as this is, it also provides the opportunity for us to widen our lens and be able to create more possibilities for respect to occur within the entire system.

In doing so, we are showing experientially the path for the members of this family to respect themselves, the other members, and the family unit with more equal balance, not one part more than another. With the awareness that self, relationships, and larger entities can be regarded as equally important and positive, respect develops more functionality and can take hold.

Case in Point

Mom (Julie) and Dad (Rick) brought in their 8-year-old son, Trevor, to talk about how Trevor should be parented. Julie begins the discussion by telling me how dangerously Rick takes risks with Trevor's well-being by insisting that Trevor play in the sports he coaches: soccer and touch football.

Dad immediately interrupts by saying that Julie is way too overly protective of their son and that she wants to have Trevor spend all of his time indoors with her, all to herself. He, Rick, never gets to spend time with his son, and he thinks that it's unhealthy for Trevor to be so tied to his mother.

Trevor is as far away as he can possibly be physically, at the far end of the couch. He is looking outside and around the room, clearly very uncomfortable being in this space. I ask him if he likes playing sports, and he nods yes, quickly looking at both parents, seeing Dad smiling broadly but Mom frowning with equal displeasure. Trevor adds in a whisper, "Sometimes I don't like it so much."

Julie pipes up, "See, he doesn't like it, Rick! He just does it because you want him to." Rick responds by saying that Julie needs to dominate everything because she is so insecure.

Trevor, squirming and trying to move even farther away, says, "No, she isn't. She's just my mommy, and she's scared I'll get hurt because she loves me. I love her too very much . . . but I won't get hurt 'cause I'm strong like my dad!"

There was further heated discussion between the parents about who was right in his or her parenting approach, both adamantly convinced that the other was harming their son. However, it became clearer and clearer that what they were really fighting over was who was getting more attention and love from their son, something that was not missed by Trevor.

He sat for a long pause after their arguing died down and then said, "I've got an idea. I'm now playing sports all weekend long, soccer on Saturdays and touch football on Sundays as well as other days in the week. Since I really like soccer better anyway, why don't I quit football, so I'm out with Dad on Saturdays and home with Mom on Sundays?" His simple compromise was genius. He had figured out his predicament in trying to please both parents who were competing for his time. He loved them both, although he was tighter with his mom because, to date, he had spent more time with her. However, he was having a blast playing sports and was getting to know his dad much better, which he really liked as well. Without knowing the words, he had intuitively realized that he was being triangulated and found, at least for now, his way out of that predicament.

The parents weren't quite as quick to pick up on this because they had more investment in keeping the triangulation going, but with more discussion about compromise and fairness to Trevor, they were able to loosen their perspectives and join their son in coming up with a workable solution. Once again, respect was the operating element that allowed for this outcome.

Groups and Transpersonal Respect

Working with groups moves the therapist into a more varied situation because the participants are unrelated and have no history with one another. The biggest initial task is to create a sense of trust and cohesiveness. Further, it is the job the group therapist to provide the understanding and respect for the individuality, the unique qualities, of each group member and the background culture that they come from. As we do so, we are also guiding the dynamics between the members such that they are also noticing their own differences and the differences of others in an honoring way. More will be said about groups in Chapter 7, but the important point here is that working with groups allows us to work with more diverse populations in which there are less-defined connections.

As this is taking place, it is hoped that there will be an expanding space to consider even larger systems, such as work and school environments, community, and more universal concepts. This expansion of the notion of respect may seem to be beyond our therapeutic boundaries or abilities, but as Thomas and Schlutsmeyer (2004) have suggested, transpersonal respect is indeed within our scope of understanding as we work with clients in that it gives a "sense of connection with the world and the many others (human and nonhuman) in it" (p. 313).

It is this transpersonal respect that holds the ideal conceptualization of humanity. Perhaps it is only occasionally that we can truly grasp it, but the more we intentionally attempt it, the more fully we can be a part of it. The more we actively participate in honoring this broader sense of humanity, the more we can offer the same participative experience to our clients.

Therefore it is from within this framework of social justice and moral conscience of inclusion that RFT can help clinicians build a foundation with our clients that maintains a specific, intentional focus on valuing human dignity and balance. Our purpose for being in this field is to alleviate mental suffering and promote wholeness in those we serve. We can do this most effectively through the lens of respect.

References

Bowen, M. (1993). *Family therapy in clinical practice*. New York: Jason Aronson.

Hendrix, H. (2007). *Getting the love you want: A guide for couples*. New York: Macmillan.

Kubler-Ross, Elisabeth. (1969). *On death and dying: What the dying have to teach doctors, nurses, clergy and their own families*. New York: Scribner.

Thomas, J. C., & Schlutsmeyer, M. W. (2004). A place for the aesthetic in experiential personal construct psychology. *Journal of Constructivist Psychology, 17*(4), 313–335.

3 Processing Disrespect
Honoring Pain and Loss

When considering our client's life experiences, we sometimes miss the most significant point. Regardless of the specific circumstances, be they physical, emotional or sexual abuse, abandonment, or other trauma, the pain and loss factors are typically at the core of the presenting problems, be they intrapersonal or interpersonal in nature. This core that affects every piece of life, this feeling of being disrespected in some significant way is often hidden or masked in a variety of ways, even to those who carry it. Not until we are able to shine some light on it, give it the fullest recognition and due respect as a very real and significant part of human experience, can we begin the healing process.

If we are willing to step into the darkness with clients, experience with them the sense of despair and suffering, then we begin the process of helping them find a flashlight, not for us to shine on them but for them to shine onto their own darkness. At first, this flashlight will seem to have no batteries, emitting no light, only accentuating the darkness, but also honoring the existing power of it. By doing so, letting the flashlight feature the darkness, the client is more able to show it to us and to perhaps see it for him- or herself a bit differently, as something separate, not quite so comingled in his or her identity, something to be revered on its own. As you both sit in this darkness, its intensity and disquieting presence create awe. Honor the power that it has. The senses can then begin to adjust. Audio, smell, taste, and touch as well as visual acclamation to the darkness begin to make it more bearable, and the flashlight can start to shine dimly, but only after such complete recognition of the darkness is fully realized by both therapist and client.

The reason for this imagery is to point out the importance of this shared understanding of the power pain holds in our lives and how respecting that power can actually work paradoxically to depower it slowly with great care. The therapist's job at this point is to help the client hold the pain safely, and express it freely, without fear of any more endangerment. No more shame, embarrassment, judgment, or disregard. The uncovering of that pain then becomes the most crucial and delicate piece of the therapeutic process to be deeply respected.

To honor the pain is not the same as honoring the behavior that pain may be exhibiting (e.g., honoring the continuation of the pattern of abuse or violence), but it is more about totally acknowledging the depth of pain and loss experienced, from which that pattern was created in the first place. Often, we encounter with clients behavior that is clearly creating more harm, such as verbal and/or substance abuse.

However, we often need to go even deeper, to the point of "looking behind the behavior," to see the person living with life-altering experiences of pain. Further, we need to have a clear path to see and comprehend the perceptions and interpretations that the painful events have created in the person's own belief constructs about him- or herself and others within the world he or she lives.

As therapists are able to develop this richer appreciation for the magnitude and weight of the pain, however that is uniquely experienced for each person, without clouding it with our own perceptions or values, we are more able to assist clients in the process of developing respectful consideration of their own pain. This is important so that they can begin to understand the impact that those hurtful experiences can have, not only emotionally but also cognitively, shaping thoughts, beliefs, and behavioral responses to life generally. If left unrecognized, these thoughts and beliefs may become rigid, perhaps subconsciously so, and potentially harmful. Helping clients begin carving out the space to be able to reconsider the way in which they carry that pain allows for a feeling of strength to shift the pain ever so slightly, making it more bearable and less dominant. It further allows for some separation between the person and the pain, such that the pain carries less shame with it for that person.

Understanding the Pain of Grief, Loss, and Trauma

The first real recognition of being respected from the client usually comes from the recognition of the therapist's depth of understanding and acceptance of the client's pain. This is often called empathy, and it is as far as feelings are regarded, but I suggest that it goes beyond that. It also requires comprehension of the thoughts and beliefs the client has about the pain and what it means in context of the rest of his or her life.

We know that the grieving process is a primary underlying theme in the therapeutic experience. Kubler-Ross (1969) offered us the greatest bulk of knowledge around this universal process of adaptation to loss or change. Whereas we most typically associate grief with death, we know that grief accompanies many life events, such as separations, divorce, moves, changes in health, and trauma.

The more we can help clients honor their grief as a healthy response to painful events and walk with them through some of that grief, the more we allow them to process it in the way they most need, without judgment. All or some of the Kubler-Ross stages of grief may appear in various orders and time spans as they need to occur for each individual. It is important to allow each person to be the driver of his or her own journey.

In my 40 years as the therapist, I've come to realize that sitting with clients' pain for extended times is one of the more difficult challenges in this work and yet one of the most significant things we can do. We all wish for the chance to rush in and relieve the pain for ourselves as well as the client. But the more seasoned we become to the whole process, we will, it is hoped, become more comfortable in allowing the expression of pain to exist and understand the wisdom in doing so. It is in the silence that honoring the pain becomes the most profound. We, in that moment, allow clients the chance to move on.

Case in Point

Bobbie, a 42-year-old Caucasian woman, lost her 17-year-old son to cancer. She had gotten divorced 2 years prior and lost her aunt, who had for the most part raised her, 9 months prior to her son's death. Bobbie was an educated businesswoman and had always felt in control of her life as she managed her staff team and her family life. The divorce began the unraveling of her smoothly operated world because she had not expected it. She reflected later that she was ultimately feeling relieved because there had been a great tension in the marriage for a long time.

Losing her aunt had been more painful because she had been the only "real mother " Bobbie ever had, but she was 87 in a nursing home and had Alzheimer's for years, so Bobbie had made peace with that loss and was moving on.

Her son, Scott, however was an entirely different matter. He had been very involved with sports, a football player, a smart and a very charming young man, and the love of her life. When he was diagnosed with leukemia 6 months ago, Bobbie took charge, taking him to the best doctors in another city and staying up late many nights reading everything she could about the best-known treatments, both traditional medical treatments and alternative treatments. No money was spared when it came to his care. But the cancer was so advanced when it was diagnosed; it progressed very rapidly and was fatal.

Bobbie crashed into total devastation. She had lost her reason for living, she said. She took all the bereavement time and vacation and sick time off from work, essentially coiled up in her bed, not eating or sleeping, so deeply depressed she didn't know day from night.

She made it into my office with the help of a neighbor, 3 days before all her leave was up, to get a letter for an extension. She was clearly despondent, but with the neighbor's help, I was able to get her agreement to come back the next week. For the next several months, she and I sat with her tears, woeful wales, and long silences until she was able to start verbalizing her deep pain. She expressed never feeling anything like this before and yet also feeling numb to every-thing at the same time. Slowly came the pictures and the memories of his childhood. The anger at his lost adulthood burst frequently. I explained to her that losing a child is a form of complex grief that takes more time to heal because it is out of the natural order for young ones to die first. She heartily agreed, saying how guilty she felt, outliving him.

Time passed, the degree of pain diminishing by only hundredths of a centimeter at a time. But she was able to eventually go back to work. Friends, neighbors, and coworkers became more important to her as she realized the support they could be. She left therapy knowing that her pain was honored and respected and that she could honor it and begin to respect herself again. Therefore, she could move toward let-ting go of little pieces of the pain, allowing life to be more manageable and eventually once again worthwhile.

Grief and trauma, often overlapping—the devastating event(s) that happen during a person's lifetime, such as severe loss, abuse, or abandonment—are probably the most predominant underlying causes for persons seeking coun-seling, other than major mental health disorders. PTSD, that which comes after such trauma, can manifest in many different ways, depending on the source(s) and severity or longevity of the trauma (Horowitz, 1997). Initially, PTSD was most notably identified with combat as it was first recognized by the military dealing with veterans coming home from war zones. We now recognize that there are more widely experienced forms of trauma, includ-ing childhood abandonment, physical and sexual abuse, unexpected losses through suicide or murder, natural disasters, and so forth. It is particularly evident in clients who have endured sustained and/or multiple occurrences of traumatic events (Herman, 1992). In addition to the classically identified symptoms of PTSD, we now understand that trauma, especially experienced in childhood, can and often does create attachment difficulties or disorders later on in people's lives. Understanding the significance of attachment as it relates to mental health is somewhat new in the field, although some would say that the connection could be traced back to Freud (Johnson, 2003).

Attachment and Respect

Attachment theory has been developing over decades, originating from the work of Bowlby (1988). It has been disputed as to its validity until recently as more evidence-based credibility has emerged, as cited by Johnson (2003):

> Bowlby's emphasis on emotional accessibility and responsiveness and the necessity for soothing interactions in all attachment relationships, once so unfashionable, is now supported by empirical work such as studies on the nature of distress in marital relationships.
>
> (p. 4)

The recognition of a universal need for attachment, and the lack thereof, substantiates the assertion put forth by RFT that respectful, positive connection with others is necessary for healthy personal growth. Attachment even further suggests that these connections need to be meaningful and foundational in terms of creating a solid base for self-respect and the ability to truly develop sound, respectful relationships with others.

To this point of establishing a foundation for healthy bonding in the future, Johnson (2003) suggested:

> It is this need, and the fears of loss and isolation that accompany this need, that provide the script for the oldest and most universal of human dramas that couple and family therapists see played out in their offices every day.
>
> (p. 4)

Going a step further, Bowlby (as cited by Johnson) talks about the overconcern we have about dependency: "Dependency, which has been pathologized in our culture, is an innate part of being human rather than a childhood trait that we outgrow" (p. 5).

This is a critical point: that dependency of any kind, under any circumstances, can and often does carry such negative connotation and judgment rather than being seen as a basic component of just being alive. Clarifying, Johnson said:

> There is only effective or ineffective dependence. Secure dependence fosters autonomy and self-confidence. Secure dependence and autonomy are thus two sides of the same coin, rather than dichotomies. . . . The more securely connected we are, the more separate and different we can be.
>
> (p. 5)

So, assuming that identified trauma can and does create a break in secure attachment, I believe that it is an essential piece of the healing process for both therapist and client to develop a deeper respect for the pain as well as its source. This requires patience and the ability to sit with the pain, giving full permission to the client not to close or conceal it but to fully express it without shame. Sharing that deep respect for the darkest of events and all the emotions, thoughts, and beliefs surrounding them lifts the life experience up to a place that is a little more bearable and manageable. As this process continues, we begin the journey with our client through mutually honoring the pain to slowly diminish that pain and honor the entire self even more.

Case in Point

Ray, a 52-year-old Caucasian male, reported a long history of family incest and abuse, starting from his earliest memory at age five, watching his father rape his older sister, age 12, who became pregnant as a result. His father later molested Ray as well. He eventually went to prison for both acts. The adolescent Ray, who had a short temper as a result of this double trauma, was later convicted of assaulting a young man who he said looked a lot like his father. Ray spent time in juvenile detention and probation for 5 years.

Several years later, Ray got married and started his own family. His wife divorced him after 12 years of marriage because she said she caught him hurting their 8-year-old daughter. He denied it, as did the daughter, and no proof could be found, but in the divorce decree, he was denied any visitation with her nonetheless because it was a "he said, she said" situation.

He came to see me because his lawyer told him the only way to have a prayer of seeing her again was to go to counseling. The chances were pretty slim, said the lawyer, but he actively pursued it, telling me that he "just wanted to make things right."

Over the course of the next few months, he was able to tell me his life story, which was obviously excruciating for him. He talked about his childhood in a very detached, reporter-like, yet physically tense style, even about his own episode of being molested, but he refused to talk about anything to do with his sister.

It took several more sessions of building trust, allowing him the opportunity to approach his unbearable pain with more respect and compassion, before he was able to address his memory of watching sister's nightmare. He then froze in a heavy sweat, until he finally released the first tears, with many more to come.

It was this very first episode of watching the cruelty done to his sister that so filled his existence with shame and guilt that he was emotionally paralyzed, unable to feel anything about the events that followed. My job became clearer. I needed to stay with his tears for as long as he was able to stay with and express his pain. As he confronted his haunting horror, seeing such brutality as a young child, and the overwhelming guilt accompanying that event, he was able to release a huge stumbling block for his healing.

Recognizing his powerlessness in that situation as a child and forgiving himself for being powerless freed him to be able to start regarding the rest of his life events in context. Over the next few months, we looked at each event individually, he taking responsibility for what he was able to recognize was his anger and shame around his own attempted molestation and then being falsely accused of hurting his own daughter. Forgiveness was to slowly follow, and then an integration of affirmations of his strengths, as he learned to respect himself for the first time and for his future.

Much more needed attention, no doubt, including the rebuilding of his relationship with his daughter, but respecting his need to deal with that very first and brutal trauma, as well as the violation done to him and the following sequence of life events, allowed him a way to repair his past and grow in a more positive dimension.

The Nature of Aggression

To fully comprehend the nature of trauma, it is equally important to examine the nature of the source of the traumatizing event(s), which is usually a resulting consequence of some form of aggression. Much aggression is rooted in previous trauma, perpetuating a very dangerous cycle. Therefore, it seems to me that as we study trauma and its effects on human suffering, we should also examine more intently the nature of aggression, the epitome of disrespect, and how to more effectively intercede to reduce it.

Aggression is either about survival or domination (Bandura, 1973). In the animal world, these motivations can be understood as being compatible, striving for the same end. For humans, however, it is more questionable that domination really supports survival in the true sense of preserving or protecting life.

Too often for human beings, it becomes about territorial power and control. To have that power, one must be willing and able to take power away from others. It is in that moment, in that action of taking away, that aggression becomes a negative force, for both the aggressed and the aggressor. Often fuelled by overwhelming anger, aggressive acts can have explosive and devastating effects, primarily for the victims of that action but also for the perpetrator. This becomes exponentially more harmful when multiple aggressors are involved, as in war, bar fights, mob scenes, gang fights, and so on or when one aggressor takes on multiple victims as we have too often seen at schools, places of worship, malls, theaters, work sites, and so on.

Aggressive behavior is violent as it crosses the line of respect and harm is done. Violence can take many forms, from the psychological—ridiculing, humiliating, condescending, or bullying—to becoming more dangerous, as in physical and/or sexual abuse. The emotion of anger increases the likelihood of escalated violence as it is impulsive in nature rather than thought out. If the process can be slowed such that mitigating information can be given to the perpetrator through calm, effective communication, then it becomes more possible for de-escalation to take place. This not only takes great skill from the one mitigating but some level of willingness from the aggressor. In my experience, this only is possible when respect is an active piece of the intervention.

Keeping in mind that respect means reconsideration or rethinking, it is the specific intervention needed to break the progression of aggression. For it is the cognitive, rational processing that necessarily slows the impulsive emotional behavior. The issue then becomes how to best achieve this, such that the cognitive process is allowed space to continue alongside of the emotive processing. How can newer information be helpful in understanding and responding in a way that would convey respect for self and others? It seems that any such information cannot be potentially shaming but steeped in thoughtful reflection, which lends itself toward genuine internalization of respectful insight. The therapist's role is to facilitate this availability to positive change through such reconsiderations.

So how do we bring respect into the conversation with those who show aggressive behavior without violating our own ethics by reinforcing that behavior? One obvious answer is to ask more questions about the client's thoughts and feelings about his or her own experiences of being respected or disrespected and how those experiences have impacted their lives. To first acknowledge the pain and brokenness is critical to establish safety in the whole discussion about respect. Careful to avoid any judgment, focusing on the client's sense of the damage done to him- or herself first not only establishes safety and trust, but it also provides a path into healing that broken self, which is at the very core of the work of undoing the need to harm others through aggression.

Bullies and the Bullied

Much has been written about bullying in recent decades, especially focusing on children and adolescents in school settings because that is where it is most noticeable. However, we know it can start much earlier, even in early childhood, and continue well into adulthood (Kim, Catalano, Haggerty, & Abbott, 2011). As this research suggests, childhood bullying frequently leads to violence, substance abuse, impulsivity, and poor family management in adulthood. Often, the genesis of bully behavior is in the dysfunctional familial and/or parenting style that children who bully receive. That style can be overbearing, intimidating, threatening and shaming, or physically violent. It is usually power based and stems from some previous experience with being bullied and lack of self-respect as well as respect for others. The results can be generationally devastating.

The definition of bullying has been offered in this way:

> A bully is someone who is regularly overbearing. He or she looks to cause humiliation or discomfort to another, particularly if that other is weaker or smaller. This can be physical bullying, emotional bullying or mental discomfort and humiliation.
>
> (Bullying Statistics, 2014)

Bullying most often is about imbalance of power, has intention to harm, and is repetitive. It is usually culturally based; that is, it comes out of a culture, be it familial, schoolyard, neighborhood, or workplace. Therefore it frequently is systemic rather than isolated. Addressing the larger systemic issues of bullying is a much more daunting task but usually more significant toward affecting solution-oriented change.

Case in Point

Don, a 14-year-old boy I was seeing with his family, was a quiet, polite young man in my presence. His father, a recovering alcoholic, and his mother, one to frequently rage, were near a final breakup, both blaming Don for his bad behavior in school, frequent runaways, and truancies for their marital difficulties.

I saw the family for several months with little progress. They came regularly and seemed invested in the process but also seemed deadlocked to change. Finally, the mother left the home, seemingly abandoning the family, and the sessions terminated.

A few months later, I got a call from Don. He wanted to come in individually. Transportation being a problem, he only came a few times, sporadically. But in the sessions he did attend, I learned a tremendous amount. His dad, he said was "cool" but spent little time with him. His mother, a rager, although he had a different term for her, as he reported, was constantly belittling him, blaming him for all her problems, and threatening to hurt him if he didn't shape up. He was glad she was gone.

In school there was another drama going on. He was desperately seeking friends and did not have a sense of safety with any of the teacher because he had just recently moved to that school. The peers he was attracted to happened to be gang members. He thought they were "really way cool" until one day they cornered him in the bathroom, stole his money, and told him that unless he joined their gang, they would hurt or kill his family. He subsequently did join the gang and kept his mouth shut because, he said, he was "scared to death."

> *He had a gun in his possession, which he claimed was only for pro-*
> *tection, but he really didn't want it. He wanted out of the gang, too,*
> *but didn't know how to get out. I thought about calling the police, but*
> *he had not threatened anyone, and I did not see him being of harm to*
> *others. He was just a very scared boy. I gave him as many suggestions*
> *and resources as I could think of but soon lost track of him.*

For many years I have thought about Don. Scared for his safety and those around him, I've often wondered how many more like him there are in this world. It is the permeation of systemic disrespect that breeds ground for this primal need for control and power. RFT offers the givers and receivers of painful interchanges similar reconsideration to aid their process of like reconsideration, such that they will learn to respect themselves and others more. The overlying problem of an ongoing generational, systemic, and social issue still exists. But therapists can take small, collective steps toward reducing this dysfunction by helping the client replace it with healthy doses of respect.

Abusive Relationships

In cases of domestic violence as well as sexual abuse, we concentrate our focus on the safety and well-being of the victims of the abuses because it is there that the most harm is done. The trauma is severe, and they are most vulnerable for potential further harm. This abusive trauma very often becomes cyclical, even a way of life for both in this relationship, because of the interdependence that becomes codependence rather than true intimacy.

Hayes and Jeffries (2016) conceptualize domestic violence as a form of terrorism and further suggest that it is much more pervasive than political terrorism with substantially less notice. They further assert that such violence is truly all about coercive control, which they define in this way: "Coercive control is a pattern of intentional tactics employed by perpetrators with the intent of governing a woman's (or man's) thoughts, beliefs or conduct and/or to punish them for resisting their regulation" (p. 3).

Given this assertion of intentional control, the real danger for therapists is to get pulled into blaming the victim in any way, especially assuming that this person could leave if he or she really wanted to. The dynamics in this kind of relationship are so complex and multilayered that it is not prudent or respectful to come to such simplified solutions.

The typical stages of domestic violence and cycle fairly predictably are the following:

- Abuse—the lashing out, belittling, harmful behavior that is done to be a show of power and control
- Guilt—not necessarily remorse for the behavior but fear of consequences

- Excuses—rationalizations and blaming the victim
- "Normal" behavior—trying to maintain the relationship, acting as nothing happened and/or gas-lighting, or putting on the charm
- Fantasy and planning—ruminating over wrongs he or she perceives in the victim and planning the next abusive episode
- Set up—setting the stage, creating a situation that from the abuser's perspective, is just cause for more abuse

(HelpGuide, 2014)

Many factors such as fear of safety risks, for oneself or for children, financial instability, or the psychological damage already done to the victim as well as what is assured to continue, create a devastating erosion of personal power and confidence. This can contribute to the stalemate position often felt by the victim.

Case in Point

Bob and Jennifer had originally come in to see me for "communication issues." They had been together for 7 years, married for three. They had one daughter, age four. Bob had been married twice before, was 10 years older than Jennifer, and had two teenage children, whom he claimed had "abandoned" him, due to the "brainwashing" of their respective mothers.

In our first session, Jennifer was very quiet, looking down at her lap or turning her head away from both Bob and me as Bob was doing most of the talking in a very charming way. He was telling me how concerned he was about his wife because she was so despondent. As he explained, "She sleeps all the time, doesn't cook or clean the house, and sometimes doesn't even bathe!" As I looked at her, she had a flood of tears rolling down her cheeks, but would not speak, and turned herself even further away from us.

Trying to get more history information, I asked Bob how long this had been going on and if there was any pattern to this behavior. As he started to speak, she suddenly turned toward us and glared at me and then at him. He stopped speaking and stared back at her with an instantly enraged appearance. I attempted to de-escalate the two of them by suggesting that it was commonly difficult in the first session to talk about these kinds of raw feelings, and it was OK for them to take their time. After a few moments of silence, I asked Jennifer if she had anything to say, but she declined. I didn't push it.

As the weeks went on, the sessions were sporadic. When they did come in, Bob seemed more and more agitated, especially when she began to speak. Finally, he quit coming. She did too, for a while, but eventually came back. The stories she told me, I had expected. They were about Bob controlling the money, her limitations on friends, and his outbursts when she did clean, but not to his liking, the name-calling and, yes, the occasional push, shove, or slap. She was most terrified of his really loud, booming voice that would seem to come from nowhere. She was also afraid for her daughter. She had thought about leaving several times, but had no money, and was terrified of his reaction if she took her daughter, whom she would not leave behind. Besides, she described, he calmed down after each episode, actually, and was loving toward her and the child for a little while.

During these early sessions with her, I just listened to her immense pain and allowed the space for her to process through the various layers of pain that she had been holding in so tightly. Fear had been dominating her life for so long that she could not recognize how much agony she was experiencing. As she permitted herself to express her depth of hurt, anger, even disgust, with the situation she found herself in, she gradually was able to see it more fully and begin to separate her self-identity from it.

We will be considering this part of the process, separating self from the pain, in the next chapter, but the necessary first step of understanding and appreciating the power pain holds over the person is the most critical. In many cases this is the most difficult piece of the process for the client. We need to be keenly aware of this and take our time and utmost care in moving through this delicate stage.

Treating the Deep Pain of Trauma and Loss

There are a number of treatment protocols recognized for effective results with PTSD including exposure therapy, CBT, EMDR, and EFT, with some ongoing controversy about which might be most effective (Cusack et al., 2016).

EMDR is a currently recognized technique that is used for processing such trauma. Founded by Dr. Francine Shapiro in 1990, this technique is widely accepted at present to be a protocol to be used with trauma situations and is reported to be successful in many cases, as it is defined in this way: "Eye Movement Desensitization and Reprocessing (EMDR) is a psychotherapy treatment that was originally designed to alleviate the distress associated with traumatic memories" (EMDR Institute, Inc., 2016).

The clinical process and expected outcomes of EMDR are described by Shapiro, et al. (2007):

> EMDR's procedures have been developed to access the dysfunctionally stored experience and stimulate the innate processing system, allowing

it to transmute the information to an adaptive resolution, shifting the information to the appropriate memory systems.

(p. 8)

EMDR appears to be most helpful in supplementary use with other forms of therapy, such as CBT or EFT. It seems to work better for those who do not have active dissociative issues as opposed to those who are currently or recently have been abused (Paylor & Royal, 2016).

The RFT position on any specific modality is to use it wisely and to fit the modality and/or techniques within modalities to the unique needs of each client rather than the other way around. The needs of the person(s) sitting in front of the therapist should always come first. The tools that we have to work with need to be customized accordingly.

Dealing With Mental Illness

In the United States, one out of five people are dealing with mental illness every year and 60 percent of those adults and 50 percent of those age eight to 15 receive no treatment (National Alliance on Mental Illness, 2016).

The pain of this reality not only affects those who are ill but also their families, friends, loved ones, neighbors, and society at large. Because of the heartache, stigmas, and cost attached to mental illness, those who have such illnesses often are unsupported, if not forgotten, becoming homeless, often drug dependent, and/or filling up jails in record numbers. Because of a general lack of interest in effectively treating a great majority of these individuals, there tends to be a severe lack of designated public funds or insurance parity to provide appropriate mental health care and services. This population is probably one of the least valued, least respected in all humanity.

The mentally ill who are lucky enough to get any treatment, who have family to support them or other resources, often are still not adequately served. That is, they may only get medication checks once every few months and/or minimal therapy or be housed in state hospitals for years, largely because their needs are so great that they are marginalized and stereotyped as being "crazy." Often, they are overmedicated as a means of behavior control rather than given more targeted therapy to meet their specific needs.

Recovery mental health, a newer approach to working with the mentally ill, is endorsed by Substance Abuse and Mental Health Services Administration (2016): "[R]ecovery-oriented care and recovery support systems help people with mental and/or substance use disorders manage their conditions successfully" (Substance Abuse and Mental Health Services Administration, 2016).

This model addresses the need for better, more effective treatment by, offering peer specialists who advocate and support and are actively involved in the patients' lives as therapists focus more on the client's stated goals and objectives rather than those imposed by the medical staff. This approach exemplifies the tenets of RFT and has shown to be highly effective, particularly with this undervalued and frequently powerless population. Giving more control to all, including those with more severe disorders, in the process of therapy is critical in the implementation of RFT.

Mental health disorders, such as major depression, general anxiety disorder, chemical dependency, even mood and personality disorders often have their roots in post trauma as well as biogenetics. This awareness for both clinician and client further depathologizes such disorders as human responses to very difficult or horrendous experiences. If we really start to understand the scope of damage that life events have on broader human suffering, then maybe we can begin to regard persons with mental illness with greater honor and thereby unravel their suffering in more effective ways.

Addressing Addiction

Many clients who have had trauma in their lives and/or live with mental illness, for example, bipolar disorder also live with some form of addiction. This is not to say that all addiction is coexisting with these other issues. We know, for example, that chemical dependency is frequently a genetic disease. However, we also know that many people "self-medicate" with addictive behaviors. We need to be cognizant of each individual's circumstances, needs, and reasons for turning to addiction because many times they are varied and complex and may give us specific direction in how to proceed in treatment.

The life of an addict, regardless of other comorbid issues, is filled with shame and pain. Although it is intended to be self-medicating, it fast becomes a ferocious monster that disguises as a best friend. Addiction is a devastating tornado that builds from a soft, comforting wind.

Case in Point

Tim was 23 years old when he came into our CD unit. He reported in intake that he had done every kind of drug out there. Upon questioning, the staff could not find him wrong; he had indeed taken every drug they named, and this was verified through his UD.

In those days we ran a standard 28-day program. Tim was actively working with the program in the first week, which was pretty unusual because denial and anger typically precede, especially during the detox stage and even more especially when that detox involves so many varied chemicals. But Tim was convincing in his ongoing statements that he didn't want to die and he knew he would soon if he didn't do something about it now.

We found out that week that Tim had been on the street for months, pimping his money for drugs. He had left home at 15 because his father was a raging alcoholic and was scapegoating Tim, blaming him for his parents' divorce. He had been in jail twice, once for intoxication and possession and the next for pimping, although his lawyer got him off with a lighter sentence.

We were initially puzzled by his intense interest in sobriety, especially so early in treatment because that level of interest usually doesn't occur until after detox and then weeks or months into sobriety. But then he shared in group one day that he hated his father's drinking so badly that he'd promised himself in second jail lock-up that he would never repeat this pattern again.

Unfortunately, Tim was kicked out of treatment early, and I was sure that he would be back using that night and dead by the end of the month. However, to my elated surprise, several months later, I saw him in a restaurant, and he reported that he had stayed sober from that day of hospital release and was now chairing a Narcotics Anonymous group.

I went home that night with such a sense of awe that anyone with such a history of dysfunction, trauma, and addiction could be strong enough to, indeed, move forward with his life in such a courageous way. Addiction is such a mean disease, ruining so many lives, and is usually accompanied by trauma and dysfunction, that I am honestly humbled by those who commit to and stay in recovery.

Those who work in our field with addiction often become somewhat discouraged in the process of recovery because it so often is pelted with relapses. But staying open to possibility, as well as earnestly honoring the pain underneath, keeps us engaged and most helps clients move on their paths forward.

Self-Harm and Suicide

Perhaps the deepest level of emotional pain that we see is exhibited through acts of self-harm and suicide attempts or, at worst, completion. Self-harm includes addictive behaviors, eating disorders, and cutting or burning behaviors. Most literature suggests that typically these behaviors are related to childhood trauma and PTSD (Low, Jones, MacLeod, Power, & Duggan, 2000).

The pain inflicted on oneself is representative of the inner psychological pain that the person is holding. To be able to deeply respect that pain, even when it appears to be self-inflicted and perhaps mostly for attention-seeking purposes, is to honor that person's reality as they are experiencing it in the moment. This is not to say that we support self-injurious behavior but that we honor the intensity of the thoughts and feelings that sit behind that behavior.

The ultimate danger in self-harm is the risk potential for suicide. Suicide is the 10th-leading cause for deaths in the US, and 90 percent are caused by some form of mental illness, including PTSD (National Alliance on Mental Illness, 2016).

Suicide is by far the most devastating of outcomes as it reflects the apex of human misery. The person who attempts or completes suicide, on purpose or accidentally, is making the strongest statement of his or her pain and that statement reverberates, causing even more pain for family, friends and other support, including therapists. It is what we all most dread in this field. It signifies complete loss of hope and ultimately, a failure to respect one's own humanity. This is one of the most definitive reasons that RFT is so vital to maintain: to reconstruct the element of respect in people's lives.

References

Bandura, A. (1973). *Aggression: A social learning analysis*. Prentice-Hall.

Bowlby, J. A. (1988). *Secure base: Clinical applications of attachment theory*. London: Routledge.

Bullying Statistics. (2014, December 27). Parents that bully children and more. Retrieved from http://www.bullyingstatistics.org/content/bullying-parents.html

Cusack, K., Jonas, D. E., Forneris, C. A., Wines, C., Sonis, J., Middleton, J. C., . . . & Weil, A. (2016). Psychological treatments for adults with posttraumatic stress disorder: A systematic review and meta-analysis. *Clinical Psychology Review*, *43*, 128–141.

EMDR Institute Inc. (2015, November 1). What Is EMDR? Retrieved from http://www.emdr.com/what-is-emdr.html

Hayes, S., & Jeffries, S. (2016). Romantic terrorism? Survivor narratives of psychological and emotional tactics of domestic violence. Stop Domestic Violence Conference, 7–9 December 2015, Canberra, A.C.T.

HelpGuide (2014). Domestic violence and abuse. [12/22/2014], Retrieved from (http://www.helpguide.org/articles/abuse/domestic-violence-and-abuse.htm#cycle

Herman, J. L. (1992). Complex PTSD: A syndrome in survivors of prolonged and repeated trauma. *Journal of Traumatic Stress*, *5*(3), 377–391.

Horowitz, M. J. (1997). *Stress response syndromes: PTSD, grief, and adjustment disorders*. New York: Jason Aronson.

Johnson, Susan M., & Whiffen, Valerie E. (Eds.). (2003). *Attachment processes in couple and family therapy*. New York: The Guilford Press.

Kim, M. J., Catalano, R. F., Haggerty, K. P., & Abbott, R. D. (2011). Bullying at elementary school and problem behaviour in young adulthood: A study of bullying, violence and substance use from age 11 to age 21. *Criminal Behaviour and Mental Health*, *21*(2), 136–144.

Kubler-Ross, Elisabeth. (1969). *On death and dying: What the dying have to teach doctors, nurses, clergy and their own families*. New York: Scribner.

Low, G., Jones, D., MacLeod, A., Power, M., & Duggan, C. (2000). Childhood trauma, dissociation and self harming behaviour: A pilot study. *British Journal of Medical Psychology*, *73*(2), 269–278.

National Alliance on Mental Illness. (2016, January 31). Mental Health Facts in America (n.d.) Retrieved from https://www.nami.org/NAMI/media/NAMIMedia/Infographics/GeneralMHFacts.pdf

Paylor, S., & Royal, C. (2016). Assessing the effectiveness of EMDR in the treatment of sexual trauma. *The Practitioner Scholar: Journal of Counseling and Professional Psychology, 5.*

Shapiro, F. (2007). EMDR and case conceptualization from an adaptive information processing perspective. In *Handbook of EMDR and family therapy processes*, Kaslow, F. and Maxfield, L. (Eds.). Hoboken, NJ: John Wiley & Sons, 3–34.

Substance Abuse and Mental Health Services Administration. (2016, January 29). *Results from the 2014 National Survey on Drug Use and Health: Mental Health Findings*, NSDUH Series H-50, HHS Publication No. (SMA) 15–4927. Rockville, MD: Substance Abuse and Mental Health Services Administration.

Substance Abuse and Mental Health Services Administration. (2016). Recovery and Recovery Support (n.d.) Retrieved from http://www.samhsa.gov/recovery

What is EMDR?, EMDR Institute Inc. (2015, November 1) Retrieved from http://www.emdr.com/what-is-emdr.html

4 Rebuilding the Self
Growing Into Personal Respect

Recognizing and fully honoring the pain in the client's life experience is the first and perhaps the most significant step we can take, requiring intense work and time for both therapist and client. At times it may seem as though this is as far as we can go in the process because that pain is so pervasive.

However, it is our obligation to help the client proceed into the next phase, healing and regaining a sense of personal respect. This is when respect from the therapist is so pivotal, such that clients might begin to find the ability to respect themselves again, if not for the first time. This phase of individual therapy concentrates on rebuilding the damaged parts of a person, damaged by trauma, shame, or loss. It helps clients see themselves in more positive ways, demonstrated through self-forgiveness, finding a path toward acceptance, meaning, and purpose.

Moving in this direction is also rigorous and slow, depending on the severity of the client's needs. Following the recognition of pain and shame is movement toward self-forgiveness, and affirmation of self, slowly giving way to a deeper, more substantive respect for one's dignity, integrity, and core values. It takes courage to become vulnerable and authentic (Brown, 2012), but this is essential to the undertaking of redefining oneself positively. Although this journey is fluid and ongoing through a lifetime, the person injured can create a firmer sense of self, which supports his or her resiliency as they move forward.

Personal Respect Versus Self-Esteem

Much has been researched and written about self-esteem, yet comparatively little has been done on the issue of self-respect (Kristjánsson, 2007). For example, Shapiro (1984) suggests that self-esteem is based on a sense of autonomy or self-sufficiency. However, Kristjánsson asserts that self-esteem seems to be more about how one feels about oneself, based upon achievements or mastery of skills, such as those found in academics, professions, sports, and so on or in roles or status in life—this is, a parent, wife, husband, CEO, and so on—all of which can be noted and confirmed by others.

He also notes that there is global self-esteem, an overall esteem for oneself, as well as domain specific.

Nonetheless, Kristjánsson makes the case that both are ultimately inadequate because esteem is about external, temporal appreciations of oneself instead of internal, consistent valuing of one's core values, dignity, or integrity. Further, he contends that self-respect should replace self-esteem, because

> [m]any ethicists complain—the concept of self-esteem lacks an objective moral grounding. Given that what self-esteem instruments measure is simply subjective self-reported satisfaction, amongst those individuals epitomizing high self-esteem may be the big-headed bully, the smug drug baron, and the Machiavellian tyrant (p. 225).
>
> (cf. Kristjánsson, 2007)

RFT also postulates that self-esteem without respect is too shallow and that the addition of respect creates a more solid positive foundation. Instead of replacing esteem, however, RFT contends that respect for oneself builds upon some already established esteem. Attempting to help build personal respect without addressing esteem issues first is much more difficult.

Personal respect, then, is a deeper understanding of oneself, with greater internal valuing. It is solid and ethically grounded. Figure 4.1 illustrates the differences and how the two concepts interrelate.

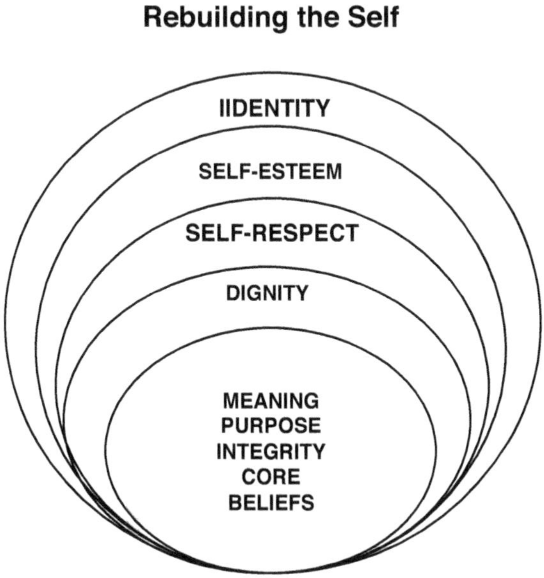

Rebuilding the Self

IIDENTITY

SELF-ESTEEM

SELF-RESPECT

DIGNITY

MEANING
PURPOSE
INTEGRITY
CORE
BELIEFS

Figure 4.1 Rebuilding the Self

Self-esteem is here shown to be an externally based set of experiences. Often it's about gaining approval from others and therefore allows for more appropriate social behaviors. Narcissism can distort that esteem in ways that Kristjánsson previously described, but in healthier circumstances esteem can boost confidence by providing some motivation for functioning in relationship to others. It also provides some protection from the negativities encountered in the environment.

However, it is respect for oneself that actively carries one's dignity, integrity, and core beliefs as well as purpose and meaning. Respect for one's own interior as a whole being is much more substantial and sustainable if it is authentically held with honor and reverence. A person with genuinely rooted respect is able to hear criticism constructively. In fact, it is those with well-developed respect for themselves who are best able to process criticism analytically, discern that which may be useful, and use it productively, correcting their own beliefs, actions, or direction in ways that improve life quality.

Given the level of damage done to the individuals we typically see in the therapy room, it is common that we encounter people who have profound deficiencies in self-respect. This is a primary premise in the RFT framework. Yet it is also central to RFT to assume that in the innermost interior of all human beings, there is, in fact, the capacity to find and connect with a true sense of core respect for oneself, be it hidden far beneath the hurt and related shame. Our principle role as therapists is to aid in the process of grounding in genuine self-respect. As the negative beliefs and feelings are countered with the development of respect, positive feelings and perspective spark interest in further nurturing what lies deeper inside.

Dignity

According to Aharon Barak, human dignity is a constitutional human right (Coffey, 2016). This is not a scorecard or rating system of our personal worthiness. Instead, it is genuine acceptance and love for our very existence. Social prejudices and interpersonal trauma, such as rape or incest, can rob us from such a secure position. Reestablishing our dignity comes through the work we do to invoke self-respect.

It is about becoming aware of the fact that we not only have the right to exist but that we have real value in our existence. Dignity allows us to own who we truly are: imperfect yet complete beings. With our dignity restored, we can be scarred, even disgraced by life events, but still carry a sense of solidarity within that no external factors can subtract from us.

Respect plays a key part in establishing and maintaining such dignity. It holds one's dignity in place and keeps it fully operational for the purpose of self-determination. That determination allows us the freedom and power to make decisions and judgments in our own best interests rather than forfeiting that power to others. Dignity does not preclude the opportunity for growth; instead it actively welcomes all avenues for becoming the best we can be. It allows us to embrace that which is good in us: our integrity, meaning, and purpose.

Integrity and Self-Forgiveness

Integrity is that part of ourselves that holds us accountable to our core beliefs and is at the heart of respecting who we really can be. This accountability includes a standard in human behavioral values but should not be so rigid as to make that standard humanly unachievable. No one is above making mistakes or bad choices. Our sense of well-established integrity, therefore, necessarily includes compassion, forgiveness, and grace.

The pathway to achieving such a balance of morality and the ability to genuinely forgive one's perceived shortcomings are frequently interrupted or broken by trauma and the resulting life experiences, such as PTSD, addiction, depression, or other mental impairments. As we will see in the case study presented in this chapter, integrity may seem as if it is unattainable or out of one's reach even as it is already there.

Shame often becomes a dominant source of blockage around the trauma(s), and the resulting experiences or behaviors by the traumatized or impaired, because it frequently becomes the way we interpret those negative events in our lives. We tend to internalize those events and cast blame on ourselves. Therefore, self-forgiveness becomes key to repairing the psychological damage done by shame.

According to Bauer et al. (1992), "[T]he structure of self-forgiveness, or more accurately that of 'experiencing forgiveness' involves a shift from fundamental estrangement to being at home with one's self in the world" (p. 153). These authors emphasize that the phenomenon of self-forgiveness is experienced as a gift, not as an achievement in isolation, but in context of being with others. Halling, Leifer, and Rowe (2006) add, "[T]he moment of forgiveness appears to be the moment of recognition that it has already occurred. . . . Forgiveness comes as a revelation and is often viewed as a gift" (p. 258).

The layers of one's own guilt, justly assessed as such or not, mixed with familial shame or collective shame of others, such as being a soldier in combat and observing death and destruction, can literally take years to sort out.

As Hall and Fincham (2005) point out, the research literature on self-forgiveness is sparse in comparison to that on interpersonal forgiveness, but they have similar properties, which are necessary for true personal respect to be achieved:

> Few definitions of self–forgiveness can be found in the social science literature, but those that do exist emphasize self–love and respect in the

face of one's own wrongdoing. . . . Similarly, Holmgren (2012) argues
that in self–forgiveness, the offender recognizes his/her intrinsic worth
and its independence from his/her wrongdoing.

(p. 623)

This process of self-forgiveness, then, is not about making excuses for one's
behavior but truly acknowledging wrongdoings done with grace, letting go
self-imposed penalties, self-regret, hatred, or other forms of disregard. It is
also about being able and willing to make amends and correcting hurtful
behavior where and when possible in context of relating to others (Halling,
2006).

Margaret Holmgren (2012) writes more about self-forgiveness as it
relates to self-respect. She asserts:

The first task for the wrongdoer (self) is to recover enough self-respect
to recognize that she is a valuable human being in spite of what she
has done. Without self-respect, it is unlikely that she will be able to
accomplish any of the other tasks involved in responding to her own
wrong.

(p. 76)

The correlation between self-respect and self-forgiveness then seems to be
made clear. They are interdependent; one does not appear to be fully viable
without the other. It then makes the therapeutic process necessarily inclusive of both goals.

Meaning and Purpose

As we develop or restore these more significant, or sacred, if you will, parts
of our innermost selves, we come to recognize that there is even more to be
discovered within our existence. Existentialists such as Victor Frankl and
Rollo May have written at length about meaning and purpose. For at some
point, there has to be more than just acceptance of self; it seems that we also
need a reason for existing. That reason for many is spiritual in dimension;
for others it can be about family, vocation, or cause, but in any regard, we
all need some sort of purpose and meaning to drive us forward.

Victor Frankl is perhaps one the most famous leaders in the discussion
of meaning. In his signature book, *Man's Search for Meaning*, he talks
about his many years as a prisoner in Auschwitz, where mere survival was
the source of meaning, and yet in such a deplorable setting, the search for
further meaning became even more important. In this book he says, "[S]triving
to find a meaning in one's life is the primary motivational force" (2006,
p. 99).

Later on in life, after his freedom from the concentration camp,
Frankl, who was a psychiatrist, developed a model for therapy, known

as logotherapy. The Greek word *logo* actually means "meaning" so that logotherapy is an existential therapy that particularly focuses on assisting persons work on their search—or will—for meaning. He speaks frankly about such will:

> Man's will to meaning can also be frustrated, in which case logotherapy speaks of "existential frustration." The term "existential" may be used in three ways: to refer to (1) existence itself, i.e., the specifically human mode of being; (2) the meaning of existence; and (3) the striving to find a concrete meaning in personal existence, that is to say, the will to meaning.
>
> (pp. 100–101)

Joseph Fabry (1980), a prodigy of Frankl's, wrote more about logotherapy, saying, "Logotherapy. . . draws our attention to the storehouse of specifically human resources within ourselves on which we can rely to restore and maintain our mental health" (p. xiv). He then points out that there are two different levels of meaning, universal and individual. About universal meaning, he states, "As ultimate meaning, a universal order in which every person has a place . . . the search for meaning raises questions as to our identity, purpose, direction, and tasks" (p. xv). In contrast, he offers a more personalized concept of meaning by saying, "Each person is a unique individual going through a sequence of unrepeatable moments each offering specific meaning to be recognized and responded to" (p. xv). The point here is that we share meaning in a common universe, and we also have time specific meaning that is uniquely our own.

This is important to understand within the framework of RFT because the clinician, in his or her on belief system, may understand universal meaning differently than the client for a variety of reasons. For example, the client may not share the same worldview, that is, have the same faith base or a philosophical approach. Most everyone has a worldview, whether it is simplistic or sophisticated, optimistic, or pessimistic. Some, however, may not have a worldview fully constructed because life events have never afforded the opportunity for that construction to happen. Trauma(s) and other dysfunction have simply blocked that piece of personal development from happening. This does not imply that this person has no meaning or that they are morally deficient but simply that that particular development hasn't yet had the chance to occur. On the other hand, that person's unique meaning to time and place probably is more accessible.

To explore his or her daily sense of meaning and purpose may be a more significant starting point in this stage of therapy. For instance, one meaning may be about just getting out of bed every day and accomplishing one small task or staying sober for that day. Once some reasonable level of functionality is underway, then perhaps a more global sense of meaning can begin to occur.

It is our responsibility as therapists to try to understand where our client is in regard to his or her own concept of meaning and meet him or her at that place without judgment and with a willingness to move at his or her pace and direction in this venture.

It may seem that this depiction of dignity, integrity, and meaning are too abstract or unrealistic to implement in the therapeutic process. This is an ongoing, fluid, lifelong process that each of us grapple with daily, trying to master it. It is precisely because we as therapists are aware of our own struggles in this regard that we can better understand and respect the struggles of our clients. Every therapist is duty bound, I believe, to continue to actively work within, to maintain, and to grow one's dignity with healthy boundaries as well as nurture that same growth process in clients. It is important to maintain a sense of hope for our clients and ourselves such that growth is always possible, even in the most difficult circumstances.

Courage and Creativity in Growth

Rollo May (1980) highlights two more important components to this process: courage and creativity. Once again, respect is a verb and ultimately requires some action. For dignity, integrity, and meaning to remain vital parts of who we are, it takes courage to (re)create these ever evolving pieces of our inner self, our soul. About such courage he says:

> This courage will not be the opposite of despair. We shall often be faced with despair, as indeed every sensitive person has been during the last several decades in this country. . . . Nor is the courage required mere stubbornness—we shall surely have to create with others. But if you do not express your own original ideas, if you do not listen to your own being, you will have betrayed yourself.
>
> (p. 2)

So how does one muster this kind of courage? Where does it come from inside of us and how can we best use it to create a stronger sense of who we are and can become? I'm not sure that anyone has the complete answers to those questions, but they are valid to explore with clients as a means of starting the discussion about a new way of thinking and feeling. Creating new perspectives on our ability to have courage to move forward is a pivotal piece of the healing process. Fear and lack of confidence are obvious blocks to that process, but the more one is encouraged to entertain the notion of being courageously creative, or as Brown (2012) would put it, "Daring Greatly," the more these concepts can become useful attributes within the person.

Case in Point

Jennifer, whom we met at the end of the last chapter, had initially come into couple counseling with her husband, Bob. After a few sessions it became apparent that that she was afraid of Bob, who was loud and displayed controlling behavior in session. After Bob quit coming because it became obvious to him that he could not control the sessions, Jennifer started coming in on her own.

She then slowly started telling me more of her story, which not only included a pattern of abuse from Bob but a much longer pattern of abuse from ex-boyfriends as well as her father, uncle, and brother, each of whom had been either physically or sexually abusive and extremely emotionally abusive as well. Her mother did not or could not protect her during her childhood because she had also been chronically abused, depressed, and alcohol dependent.

Needless to say, Jennifer had a very negative view of herself. Fear and shame dominated her life. Shame was the result of repeatedly being told by most of her abusers and her mother on occasion how stupid and worthless she was, feeling devalued and humiliated by her sexual abusers and broken physically and emotionally by the violent battering done to her over most of her lifetime.

So, the work ahead of us was one of navigating through all the various levels of pain in her past and present, giving full recognition to each piece as it was revealed, but then also starting to help her separate her identity from her pain. This process is not linear; it is necessarily woven into the healing process with the goal of becoming more singularly important as the intensity of the pain recedes.

The complexity of Jennifer's emotional, psychological, and physical injuries were not only multiple in count but also chronic in terms of creating a lifelong pattern of victimization, along with a negative view of herself. She had attempted suicide twice; the second time was almost successful and had scared her so badly that she said she would not try it again, although she admitted to thinking about it daily. She also admitted to drinking three to four glasses of wine a day and smoking pot at least twice a week. She had been in jail three times: twice for possession of illegal substances and once for prostitution, a gig her wonderful husband, Bob, had set up.

When describing herself, she would use words like "slut," "whore," and "no-good trash." As we discussed her depiction of herself, I would occasionally challenge her by asking more about what she meant by using those terms, how long she felt they had actually applied to her, and what it might be like if she could substitute those words for less-offensive words like "imperfect" or "flawed." At those points she would laugh at me and several times asked me, "And who's the crazy person in the room?" I would chuckle back, acknowledge she may have a point, but then softly ask again if she could come up with any less-denigrating descriptions of herself. At first I would only get angry outbursts like, "How f-ing stupid are you? If I had any other words that fit me, I wouldn't be here! I'm just wasting my time. None of you people (counselors) get it!" Frequently she would run out of the room but usually came back in before the time was up for that session.

I knew this was going to be a very slow-moving process. I was intentional about not getting rattled and always thanked her for coming back. I often noted her bravery in sticking with this and how difficult this must be for her, which she often scoffed at. But I could see the tiniest grin, covered as a twitch, when I made such comments.

Weeks went by with little noticeable improvement. Only the fact that she kept coming gave me hope that she had any interest in finding those other words. I volunteered several dozen, none of which were approved by her. Early on, I had asked her to keep a list of positive words or thoughts she had during the week, an assignment that had not materialized at all and I considered an aborted mission.

In the meantime, I had been focusing with her on the power of the words and actions of others and on how she had very little choice about internalizing their demolishing affects. How could anyone who had been so degraded for so many years—yes, most of her life—possibly come to think differently about herself? It may have seemed that I was joining her in her hopelessness, but in fact, I was echoing her pain in a way that she could feel heard yet slightly challenged to perhaps want to be heard differently. This shift took some time and was small at first, but one day after hearing me repeat this idea that it was inevitable that she was powerless to her victimization in life, she almost reflexively answered in a small voice, "But I don't have to be for the rest of my life, do I?" We sat in silence together for nearly 10 minutes, while I shook my head no and smiled at her. She trembled with silent tears. Toward the end of the session, she left saying, "I don't know, I just don't know. . . . We'll see." She stiffened back in her defensive posture, but I was pretty sure a small but significant shift had taken place.

It was obvious that she had just stuck one part of one toe in the water for only a nan-second. I truly believed that she would not show up the next week because of her fear of change. She was late for the session by about 20 minutes, but she did show. She abruptly opened my door and sat down on my couch, as though she had some very important news to tell me, but then froze in silence for several minutes. She then fumbled with her purse, pulled out a crumpled piece of paper, and gave it to me. I opened and read it and then handed it back, asking her to read it to me. She hesitated but did read the words: "I am kind." It was not a list but, much better, a simple statement of who she is versus what she is.

We obviously had a great deal of work ahead of us, but ground was now broken for us to build self-respect on. Her dignity had some framework, even though it was small and frail. I started using the word respect *with her a bit more now that there was some more reception to it.*

Initially she did not tolerate the use of the word, reverting back to "Nobody respects me, and I don't respect anyone either." I was able to point out her daughter, Kayla, asking if she respected her and if she felt respected by her. Working through the differences and commonalities of respect and love, she guessed that respect existed both ways with she and her daughter, but that was the only respectful bond she ever had. Supporting her acknowledgement of that experience, I then went a step further, asking if she expected others to respect her daughter as she grew older. This stumped her for a while because her immediate gut response was to say yes, and yet her own life experience couldn't allow her to really believe it. As she grappled with that, I started talking about basic human dignity and that every person alive deserved at least that much. She blurted out, "Oh yeah, she deserves at least that much!"

I asked her then to describe what "that much" was and why she felt her daughter deserved it. "That much" meant no one treating you like trash—not even yourself (with my prompting)—and her little girl deserved that because she was sweet and innocent. After a few minutes of letting her think about what she just said, I asked her to think about herself at that age, and might not she too deserve the same for the same reasons? Tears flooded down her face, her head shaking "no" for a good 10 to 15 minutes, then as she calmed, she very softly said, "Yes."

With that awareness of desired self-worth, and with the potential that it may exist for herself as a living human being, there was now room to explore that possibility. To assist her in that exploration, I was more focused on her strengths and competencies and openly shared that focus with her. I no longer tried to name those competencies for her but gave her space to "stumble" into them with intentional notice. For example, in her parenting, whereas she lacked consistency in discipline, she continued saying nurturing statements to and about her daughter, and as frequently as I heard them, I would comment briefly or nod my head supportively. She one day said something "kind" about her daughter and, before I could respond, said, "I really do love her, don't I?" I let her sit with that for a minute or two and then said, "Sounds like you really do." This pleased her immensely as she noted that she had never felt real love before.

With this newly established genuine attachment, I continued to draw parallels between nurturing her little one and nurturing the little girl inside of herself, the little one she once was. This parallel was initially hard to grasp, but I asked her to bring in some pictures of herself at that age. Once we examined those pictures together, she noticed how similar she looked to her daughter, and again the tears rolled down her face but with more joy this time. She did observe that the little girl in these pictures looked more sad, lonely, and scared than the ones of her daughter. I commented that this little girl, Jennifer, might need as much or more nurturing love as Kayla and that only the adult Jennifer could give her that. She gave me a stare, telling me that I was indeed the crazy one after all. After a few exchanged grins and chuckles, she said, "I only wish I could."

We worked on this idea for several weeks, and she came to the realization that she carried so much shame and hatred toward her abusers that she couldn't reach the scared little girl inside. We had already spent a great deal of time addressing the pain from each episode of abuse in her past and present, but there was another layer of healing to be done; she needed to start the process of self-forgiveness and forgiving others. I was very careful to explain that she was solely in charge of this part of her healing and that it was for her benefit only. It was to no longer be chained and powerless to the abusers and to come closer to reclaiming her self-worth, dignity, and integrity. I also pointed out that this would be a lifetime journey for her. She expressed fear and lack of confidence that she could ever do this, but she did understand the reasoning behind attempting such a feat.

During the next few months she worked diligently on this phase of her emotional recovery, journaling, writing letters to herself at different ages, including the 4-year old, which was the first memory she had of the abuse, affirming who she was at each point in her life. She then wrote to every abuser, including both of her parents—her ridiculing and physically abusive alcoholic father as well as her non-protective mother—and, finally, to her present husband Bob—releasing her anger and forgiving them each as much as she possibly could.

Bob was the most difficult one for her because he was the most present in her life.

She had thought that he was the one she most loved and trusted and, early on, had given her the love and respect she had always wanted. But he too had betrayed her, and she was now as terrified of him as she had ever been of anyone in her past.

As empowered as she was beginning to feel within herself, Jennifer still felt trapped or cursed, as she put it one day, because as much shame and anger as she was releasing from her past, more was building in her present. Bob had "forbidden" her to continue counseling months and months ago, but she had kept coming without his knowledge. When he found out, he had beaten her and taken her car keys away from her, she reported. I agreed to Skype with her because she couldn't leave her house. I pressed her to find safety with a neighbor, friend, relative, or shelter, but she was too afraid and wouldn't leave her daughter. All of her old fears were being retriggered.

At this point all I could really do was stay with her. I was feeling some frustration, after all the work we had done, that she couldn't muster the courage to leave, but I was too familiar with the pattern of abuse and the emotional entrapment imposed by the abuser—how extremely impossible it seems to get out of the way of the inevitable next storm.

In one of our Skyping sessions I asked her to consider her five best strengths and what she valued the most in her life. Of course her daughter rose to the top, but so did some interesting perspectives regarding herself. As scared as she was in her current situation, she saw herself as a survivor and a fighter. She further recognized her intelligence and ability to seek a better life for her daughter and herself. She knew she deserved more, but just didn't know how to get it. She was physically afraid of Bob and his retaliation, if she should leave.

A few days later she called me in a panic. Bob had come home drunk and started slapping her around. Kayla screamed, and Bob turned around and slapped Kayla hard. I immediately explained that I was obligated to call CPS. This initially scared her more, but as I talked more about safety, she latched on to that word. "Safety is very, very important! I've got to keep Kayla safe!" she said emphatically. We were then able to create a safety plan. She agreed to call her sister, who lived on the other side of town, and ask her to come get the two of them before Bob got home. She could stay with her for a few days and get a protective order if necessary.

As time went by I heard from Jennifer less, but she did keep me informed. She was able to get a divorce and got custody of Kayla. She stopped using all drugs and was committed to sobriety to be a better, more attentive mother. Eventually, she got a part-time job as a receptionist and got a grant to go back to school to get her CNA and later her RN degree. She wanted to give back and have a real purpose in her life.

Helping clients navigate through the rocky path of self-discovery to assert their truer identities is, in fact, our highest calling as therapists. This requires not only patience but also a finely tuned awareness of the rocks and other obstacles in that path. Additionally, we need to take great care to not create another path for them but to journey with them on the path they create for themselves, guiding them ever so slightly as to allow the smallest discoveries to build into larger ones.

As we know all too well, self-respect and respect from and toward others are quite intertwined, making the distinguishing factors between them often difficult to define. Some might say that we are a collective of the relationships we've experienced in life; others might posit that our relationships are reflections of who we are or perceive ourselves to be. In any regard, the connection exists, and it is important to be aware of this as we move forward into relational therapy. Solid self-respect most frequently rests upon secure attachments from our past and present. Our future relationships have the greatest chance of being meaningful when we bring our healthiest selves into them.

In the following chapters we will be examining respect in terms of relating to others. Specifically, we will be looking at respect as it relates to couples, families, and transpersonal relationships, that is, relating to the larger world. If we are able to take our healthier selves into these riskier interpersonal arenas, we can engage in them more successfully and promote respect more widely.

References

Bauer, L., Duffy, J., Fountain, E., Halling, S., Holzer, M., Jones, E., . . . & Rowe, J. O. (1992). Exploring self-forgiveness. *Journal of Religion and Health, 31*(2), 149–160.

Brown, B. (2012). *Daring greatly: How the courage to be vulnerable transforms the way we live, love, parent, and lead.* New York: Penguin.

Coffey, D. K. (2016). Aharon Barak, human dignity: The constitutional value and the constitutional right. *Human Rights Law Review, 16*(1), 175–176, ngv042.

Fabry, J. B. (1980). *The pursuit of meaning.* New York: Harper & Row Barnes & Noble Import Division.

Frankl, Viktor E. (2006–06–01). *Man's search for meaning.* Boston: Beacon Press.

Hall, J. H., & Fincham, F. D. (2005). Self–forgiveness: The stepchild of forgiveness research. *Journal of Social and Clinical Psychology, 24*(5), 621–637.

Halling, S., Leifer, M., & Rowe, J. O. (2006). Emergence of the dialogal approach: Forgiving another. In *Qualitative research methods for psychologists: Introduction through empirical studies,* Fischer, C.T. (Ed.) Cambridge, MA: Academic Press, 247–277.

Holmgren, M. (2012). *Forgiveness and retribution: Responding to wrongdoing.* New York: Cambridge University Press.

Kristjánsson, K. (2007). Measuring self respect. *Journal for the Theory of Social Behaviour, 37*(3), 225–242.

May, Rollo. (1980). *The courage to create.* New York: Bantam Books, W.W. Norton.

Mental health facts in America (n.d.) National Alliance on Mentally Illness. (2016, January 31). Retrieved from https://www.nami.org/NAMI/media/NAMIMedia/Infographics/GeneralMHFacts.pdf

Shapiro, D. (1984). *Autonomy and rigid character.* New York: Basic Books.

5 Interpersonal Respect
Couples Relating Respectfully

Working with couples brings more complexity and challenges. Obviously, there are two people in the room instead of one, both having their own stories of pain or brokenness. Additionally, there is the relationship between these two, which has its own brokenness. To heal the relationship, each individual must find some healing within to give functionality to the relationship. But the relationship requires more: better communication, listening skills, negotiating skills, forgiveness, and yes, respect.

Couples come into counseling because one or both individuals feel that the relationship is in trouble or needs improvement. When asked, the most common reason given in my practice experience is poor communication skills. This is, of course, a generic label put on a host of issues, which underlie the presenting complaint. The job ahead of us is clearly multidimensional.

There are two parallel processes involved with doing couple work. The first is attuning to the relationship needs, more specifically, to the presenting issues as well as related patterns of behaviors, thoughts, and feelings that contribute to those issues. Understanding the context and culture of that relationship is critical in terms of working respectfully and effectively to promote positive change. Relationships are fluid; they are changing day by day, depending on the influences of external factors and the internal realities of each person in that relationship. Therefore, this is really more complex than just the sum of two people. Attention to the evolving state of that entity called relationship requires our awareness but not to the exclusion of our continued notice of each person in the room.

Therefore, the second process, a significant parallel process, is attuning to the individual needs of each person separately. What does each individual bring into the dyad, historically and currently? What is the unique cultural context of each person's belief system and the resulting thoughts and behaviors that are actively creating the dynamics of this particular relationship? For example, how does one's experience with one's family of origin's communication style, rules, or expression of emotions affect the sense of trust in this relationship?

In both processes, the essential focus on respect becomes clear in the therapist-client relationship and, more poignantly, in the process of shifting the clients' perspectives into recognizable respect for themselves and each other. As Hendrick, Hendrick, and Logue (2010) point out:

> It seems clear that respect has been shown to be an important quality in both friendships and romantic (including marital) relationships. . . . Only recently, however, has respect been studied purposefully as an independent and important construct in romantic relationships.
>
> (p. 130)

They define the operational components of this relational respect as caring and supportiveness as well as equality and mutuality. Based on the work of Lawrence-Lightfoot (2000), who talks about the importance of symmetry in a relationship, Hendrick et al. further list resulting improvements that reflect key basic themes of respect: empowerment, healing, dialog, curiosity, as well as self-respect.

Hendrick et al. (2010) discuss two research studies that focused on the value of respect in romantic relationships and how they differed in their results based on how the studies were designed. On the first study they said, "Frei and Shaver (2002) concluded that respect appears to be an attitude held for someone based on that person's qualities . . . the 'respect worthiness' of the partner, rather than the 'free gift' of respect for a partner no matter the partner's perceived deservingness" (p. 130). Comparatively, they sited their own study, conducted fairly simultaneously, about which they said, "[U]nlike the Frei and Shaver measure, the Hendricks' scale items were not about the partner's qualities but rather about the perceptions of the respondent in relation to the partner, for example, 'I am interested in my partner as a person'" (p. 130).

This distinction will be important as we go forward considering the role of RFT in working with couples. For respect in this context is about changing the perspectives of each person toward one another rather than the evaluation of worthiness of each. As perspectives change, emotions and behaviors will follow, hopefully in more respectful ways, more as positive shifts in perspective than evaluation. Emotions and behaviors do not define a complete person but need to be seen as reactions to life events. Therefore, if someone is acting in a way that is not acceptable to the partner, then by addressing that particular behavior or set of behaviors apart from who that person is, the chance for mutual respect grows stronger. The frailty of the relationship may make this distinction more difficult for each individual to see, but as respect is woven deeper into the process, the more safety is built, making it easier to comprehend the difference. In the end, it is less about evaluation of the other and more about mutual and equal appreciation, as evidenced in thought, feeling, and behavior.

RFT and EFT

EFT had its origin in the 1980s, stemming from the earlier works of Rogers and Perl, and is closely aligned with attachment theory (Johnson, Hunsley,

Greenberg, & Schindler, 1999). The focus is clearly on affect, with the intention of "softening" the interaction the couple's experiences.

As Bradley and Furrow (2004) point out:

> Emotionally focused therapy is distinct from other couple approaches in that it places an emotional "softening event" at the core of its model of change, thereby placing priority on promoting a softened interaction. . . . (It) represents a redefinition of the relationship as one characterized by mutual accessibility and responsiveness.
>
> (p. 234)

The concept of "softening" in a relational interaction is very akin to respect in that it is allowing each person to be more vulnerable to oneself and one another. Therefore, there is greater opportunity to listen within and to appropriately attend to needs of each other. It also allows the couple to shift their perspective from a combative stance, needing to be right, to a more collaborative dialog, focusing on finding a workable solution for both. This is requisite in providing the opportunity for respect to build into the relationship.

Achieving such a shift is often one of the most challenging aspects of this process. They each bring wounds from the past, both from previous relationships, including family of origin and from within this present relationship. Understanding the multiple dimensions of the woundedness in the room will begin to unlock some of the gridlock.

Case in Point

John and Maryanne had been married for 15 years. This was the second marriage for both. They had three grown children between them.

They came in initially because they were arguing too much—at least every other day, they reported—about money, sex, and children. Maryanne was concerned that hundreds of dollars went missing each month over the past six months, and John pled innocence, claiming that she was "trying to pin everything on him." He, in turn, accused Maryanne of having a secret affair with her ex-husband, which she also denied. When I asked each of them how long they believed the missing money and the affair had been going on, they both said about 2 1/2 to 3 years. Puzzled, I asked more about what was happening at that time in their lives.

This question escalated tension and anger in the room. They both began yelling and pointing fingers at one another. They began blaming one another and one-upping each other's accusations in rapid succession, overlapping their voices such that the volume increased so significantly until no one voice could be heard. Amidst it all, I could not decipher any definitive answers to my question. This went on until I ended the session.

When they came back, two scheduled sessions later, I was able to address the level of confusion, for me, at least, in the way things had gone toward the end of our last meeting and wondered how that had felt for them. They were both apologetic, but neither one could explain what had happened or how they felt about it. They both reported that this was a typical interchange for them and that, yes, they had continued to argue in much the same way since our last session. I gently reviewed what, from my perspective, had happened in that session, reintroducing my question regarding the time period of 3 years ago. Initially met with silence, I was eventually told that Maryanne had been pregnant and had a miscarriage. I addressed the sadness and grief around that and how difficult that was for couples to cope with. There was more silence. Finally, John burst out with "It wasn't mine!"

Maryanne vehemently denied his accusation. She said that his jealousy of her ex was at the root of all their problems. She explained that her ex had been her high school sweetheart and that they had known each other since childhood, but that in their marriage, he had cheated on her numerous times, and therefore she divorced him. She added that she had since forgiven him, and although she couldn't stay married to him, they had always been good friends, still were, and probably always would be. John shot up at this point and said, "See, see, I told you she was still involved with him!" She shouted back, "You're crazy!" The race was on to see who could out interrupt, shout, and attack the other. I finally was able to quiet them and talked about listening and honoring themselves and one another. They sat for about a minute and then in almost perfect synchronization, said, "Yeah, that's the whole problem—he/she doesn't respect me!"

Weeks went by with much of this same pattern: blaming and shaming one another. It took great effort and care to create breaks in this perpetual verbal boxing match, a need to be right and to be the competitive victor. During those breaks, however, I was able to interject small suggestions of awareness of how they each were feeling and perceiving the other. For a long while my observations seemed to go unnoticed. Eventually they made a few comments like "Yea, that's exactly how I feel" or a correction, like "Well, what I really meant to say was . . ."

One day John started talking about people he could trust, unlike Maryanne. He told a story about an old buddy of his from high school who noticed that John had not bought any lunches from the cafeteria in over a week. This friend had casually offered to buy his lunch one day while they were in line going to the cafeteria. John first refused, feeling ashamed, but his friend persisted, saying that it was no big deal and that he knew what it was like not having money; he wouldn't tell anyone. John spoke about how much he felt cared about and how safe he felt in that moment. He then went on to talk about his dad, who was a chronic alcoholic and usually drank up any extra funds there might have been in the household, leaving his mom, sister, and himself without food money at all. As he told this story, Maryanne's facial and body expressions shifted dramatically. Her defensive anger seemed to melt. There was a glimpse of compassion in her eyes. As he went on with his story, John confessed that the reason money was missing every month was because he was sending that money to his mother, who still struggled to pay the bills each month, even though his dad was no longer in the picture.

He apologized for not telling Marianne about the money, but his intense shame continued to get in the way. He couldn't look at her as tears started rolling down his face. The weight in the room seemed at least 10 pounds lighter. Marianne was quiet for several minutes and finally broke into a small smile. She thanked John for his apology and then in turn apologized that he could not feel safe with her enough to tell her the truth. She admitted feeling relieved because she had thoughts of him having a gambling or drinking problem or that he was spending the money on another woman, which also made her feel unsafe.

As the sessions went on, Marianne was able to talk more about her background and how she too felt unsafe at home growing up because her mother was so verbally and sometimes physically abusive to her. Her ex-husband had become so important in her life because he provided her emotional shelter as her friend and protector. She was devastated when their marriage broke apart. When she met and married John, she thought she had found a new protector but felt very unprotected by his withdrawal and isolation. She felt safer with her ex because, with sex no longer an issue between them, he once again could be her emotional confidant.

With each of them gaining individual strength, they became better prepared to address their shared relationship. They talked a lot about trust, that is, about how hard it was for each of them but also about how much they both wanted it. They both had grown up without room to cultivate the ability to trust thoroughly. They both were afraid of it. They were going to have to learn from each other how to risk and honor their vulnerabilities.

Moving forward, we will look at ways RFT can be used conjunctively with other models of couple therapy and on its own, the interplay among respect, forgiveness, trust, and intimacy, and some cultural considerations as we honor differences with a few case illustrations.

Building Trust and Intimacy Through Respect

Trust seems to be a primary issue among couples in therapy (see Figure 5.1). As Gottman (2012) points out, "[T]rust removes an enormous source of stress because it allows you to act with incomplete information" (p. 19). In contrast, he describes betrayal as the specific source of that stress in this way:

> Betrayal is the secret that lies at the heart of every failing relationship—it is there even if the couple is unaware of it. If a husband always puts his career ahead of his relationship, then that can be another form of betrayal. When a wife keeps breaking her promise to start a family that is also betrayal. Pervasive coldness, selfishness, unfairness, and other destructive behaviors are also evidence of disloyalty and can lead to consequences as equally devastating as adultery.
>
> (p. 17)

Betrayal often is at the center of relationship discord in a variety of ways. Changing loving relational styles, including actions, words, and attitudes of warmth and support to hateful or malicious tones can constitute betrayal. Changing the understood dynamics in the relationship, that is, shifting

Relational Process With Couples

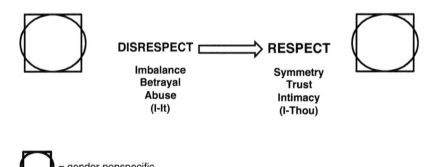

Figure 5.1 Relational Process With Couples

power or control from being equally balanced to becoming skewed or, worse, unilateral power can also result in a form of betrayal. Infidelity, of course, is the most recognizable betrayal in any relationship.

Therefore, forgiveness becomes a crucial piece in this process of building trust. As it was mentioned in the last chapter, forgiveness cannot be "forced" or "willed," but it must be freely given in such a way that the forgiver is pleasantly surprised and relieved by the removal of the anger and pain associated with betrayal. This is not to say that trust is singularly dependent on forgiveness but that both are built on openness and respect for one another.

It is also imperative to understand that both people in a relationship bring their own perceptions and expectations from not only prior relationships they have been in but also from their family of origin, the relational dynamics they witnessed from childhood, and learned patterns of behavior from their parents and other significant relatives, as Imago therapy suggests. These impressions, which often include injury such as abandonment or abuse or both, filter into the present interactions and dialog, not to mention emotional shaping within the current dyad.

So trust is built upon a multitude of factors, including current interplay between the couple but also previous experiences and culture. Culture is commonly thought of as nationality, religion, or race but also include all unique life experiences, particularly those that define our individual identities, such as sexual orientation or specific abilities and/or disabilities. Understanding how all of these influence the mechanisms of trust for each individual helps clarify the path necessary to establish such trust.

This is where respect steps in. It is not about having a complete inventory of all the contributory factors involved with one's ability to trust, but it does require an awareness of multiple influences and a willingness to suspend hurtful judgments. Respect and trust have very similar roots and necessarily comingle. Neither is based on certainty, but both require some faith in good intent. Respect in a relationship is about maintaining focus on the good of both persons, while recognizing attitudes and behaviors that need to be addressed and worked on. Trust is relying on that goodness in the relationship to be able to manage disappointments due to human error and being able to work through them as they occur.

The reality is that trust and respect need to work in tandem with one another as a unit, with both individuals engaged in the process of making this happen. In broken relationships, the divide between them usually creates asymmetry. That is, experiencing a lack of trust can reduce respect and the other way around, such that a spiral of suspicion, attempted control, and negative thoughts and feelings ensue. Our job becomes one of helping them slowly develop respect and trust as a grounded base, while the specific thorny issues are addressed. We do this with our intentional focus and by inviting them into that arena of possibility with a framework that allows them to build a healthy and safe relational bond.

This bond, then, leads the path into intimacy. Intimacy is a complex, somewhat mystifying state of being with another. Steen Halling (2008) speaks of intimacy, at least in part, to be "seeing a significant other as if for the first time" (p. 15). He goes on to say the following:

> The experience of genuinely being seen by another person is one that we deeply long for. . . . And yet we are also keenly aware that becoming visible to another is risky. . . . We go to great lengths to protect ourselves by hiding from others (and from ourselves) many of our thoughts, feelings and inclinations. Yet, while we hide, we also keep a look out for someone who might care about us and value our point of view.
>
> (p. 15)

Conversely, Halling addresses the other side of that shared experience: "[T]hat of becoming fully present to and seeing another in his or her depth and complexity . . . is an extraordinary moment in one's life and in one's relationship with the other" (p. 25). Buber's discourse on the I-Thou relationship describes the events of being intimate, particularly as it relates to couples. As Halling points out, "[T]he I-Thou relationship occurs when two people encounter each other in a radically open and mutual way" (p. 25).

Prager and Roberts (2004) echo much of what Halling says about intimacy in slightly different terms. To begin, they say, "True intimacy with others is one of the highest values of human existence; there may be nothing more important for the well-being and optimal functioning of human beings than intimate relationships" (p. 42). They follow that with the important and fundamental point that, "access to a true and authentic self is a necessary condition for intimate relating" (p. 44).

Going further in describing the tenets of intimacy, Prager and Roberts continue by saying, "[A]n intimate interaction is distinguished from other kinds of interactions by three necessary and sufficient conditions: self revealing behavior, positive involvement with the other, and shared understandings" (p. 45). Speaking specifically about self-revealing behavior, they further reinforce Halling's notion of self-protection by saying,

> Being self-revealing implies a willingness to drop defenses and invite the other to witness and to know private, personal aspects of the self. As a condition for an intimate interaction, then, some aspect of the self is willingly revealed or "exposed" to the other. Deeply self-revealing behavior usually involves the expression of emotions, and often, "vulnerable emotions" such as guilt, hurt, or sadness, that expose the "innermost self."
>
> (p. 45)

For that depth of self-revealing to occur, there must be some basis of relative certainty that there is safety in the act of showing such vulnerability.

To that point, the authors talk about the necessity of positive involvement from both partners: "For an interaction to be intimate, the individuals also need to be in a state of positive involvement. . . . Intimate relating thus precludes attacking, defensive, distancing, or alienating behavior" (p. 45). Thus, it seems that respect is an integral piece of both trust and intimacy as they are also integrated with one another. Respecting another's values, beliefs, thoughts, and feelings, especially if they differ from your own, is what allows trust and intimacy to grow and deepen.

Case in Point

Troy and Will had been living together for about 6 months. They had dated for roughly 1 1/2 years before that. They were both very skeptical of me at first, not sure that I really knew much about the gay community. Will specifically asked me if I was a Christian. When I nodded yes, Troy almost stood up as to leave. Will touched his hand, requesting him to stay, but looked equally terrified. I quickly explained that I understood the Gospel to say that I was to love and accept everyone without judgment and that I strived to live up to that without fail. I then added that I had been in practice for a long time and had the honor of working with many lesbian, gay, bisexual, and transgender (LGBT) couples and individuals over that span of time. I explained a little bit about RFT and how I use it throughout the work I do. Both men relaxed as I told them I held no judgments of them and that I had experience and knowledge related to working with their orientation and lifestyle.

Will had been in a traditional heterosexual marriage for 7 years and had a 5-year-old child from that marriage. In that marriage, they as a family had been going to a Baptist church, as Will had done growing up. He had always been taught that homosexuality was a grave sin, not to be tolerated. He was a devout Christian and had no desire to be such a sinner, but since age five had been oddly attracted to other boys. He had the same crushes on male actors and rock stars as his sisters had but dared not tell anyone, less he be laughed at and scorned. He married his best friend from college, Jean. They could laugh and cry at the same movies, enjoyed the same books, and believed very similarly in the same God. Will stated that he loved Jean very much as a good friend but was never really sexually attracted to her. He was still feeling conflicted about leaving her, especially because of their child, Tony, but he finally had found a much deeper love with Troy, even though he tried to deny it for months. He still carried much shame and guilt about it, and that was a big part of the problem that led them into my office.

Troy, on the other hand, had been openly gay since he was 15. He was from a Catholic family who were about as conservative as Will's family. But he also had an uncle who was always a closeted gay because he had been so shamed by a priest who had molested him and held him hostage to their secret by threatening to tell the whole church of his sexuality. Troy, knowing his uncle's secret, vowed never to be in the shadows. He had come out proudly and became an advocate for gay rights early in his 20s.

Will and Troy had met in a hotel bar, where Will had been for an engineer's business convention. At first they just made small talk over a basketball game on TV, but as the night went on, they huddled together at a small table and finally went up to one of their rooms and slept together. It was Will's first time to have sex with a man, although he had frequently dreamed about it. He was ecstatic but at the same time was overwhelmed by guilt. He left his convention early and went home, swearing to never see Troy again.

But that couldn't last. Try as he might, he could not stop thinking about Troy, nor could he feel any intimate closeness with his wife. He knew he was different. His whole life was different. He couldn't fake it anymore. He was gay.

Several weeks went by. He tried to pray it away. He thought about talking to his pastor but was too afraid of the repercussions. There were his good buddies at work, but he couldn't risk losing his job. He eventually started calling Troy and was so calmed and elated to hear his voice. He was, for the first time in his life, truly in love.

Having that conversation with his wife, however, went horribly. Her smile instantly changed to a look of pure hatred and disdain. She threw him out of the house immediately and wouldn't let him back in or see his son until the court-ordered visitation after the divorce. Will hated being the cause of so much pain, especially for Jean, but knew he had to move on.

Troy, on the other hand, had been out his entire sexual life. He had never had a heterosexual relationship. And admittedly, most of his relationships previously had been short-lived. This was the longest he had ever been in one. Commitment scared him, he confessed. He said the one-night-stand at the hotel was originally just that, something he was used to. But the difference was that he too had difficulty getting Will out of his head. He tried to blow it off. After all, Will was married and was uncertain of his sexual identity. Troy had been down that road before and knew it wouldn't last.

But when Will continued to call him and eventually went through a difficult divorce to be with him, he knew this was more serious. For a long while he tried to push Will away because the feelings he was experiencing "scared the hell out of him."

Will persisted and would not go away. They began dating soon after the divorce. Their courtship had been tumultuous much of the time. But they both contended that the good times outweighed the bad.

So Troy moved into Will's apartment and said he almost immediately regretted it. Will started talking about commitment and wanted to get married. And he wanted to go to church. Troy was repelled by the idea of organized religion because of what happened to his uncle, and he didn't see the point of marriage, especially as there was no legal gay marriage in the state where they lived. Furthermore, Troy's parents had split before he could talk; he had seen his father exactly twice after that, and both of those times there was a violent scene between his parents with the cops called. His mother had a long list of men who revolved in and out of their lives. Most of them were abusive to him and/or his mother, and concerning the ones who were relatively nice to him, he dare not get close to because they would leave soon.

So the dialog that typically happened in my office between the two went something like this: Will would begin by telling Troy how much he loved him and wanted to be with him always. Troy would smile broadly until he heard the word always. *He would quickly become disgruntled and defensive. "There you go, expecting the moon from me! I can't live in your Hollywood world!" Will would become sullen and say, "But I gave up my Hollywood world for you." And then they were off and running, blaming and shaming each other as fast as they could, not hearing anything the other one said.*

After several weeks of what I call "the blame and shame game," I stopped them and quietly urged them to listen and pay attention to what the other one was saying. I then asked them to do something I knew they would find uncomfortable. I explained the exercise of active listening. One person has the floor for 3 minutes, while the other may not speak, and then the other repeats what the first one said as closely as possible without comment but getting clarifications from the first for accuracy of the message received. And then the process is reversed.

The first time they tried it, the outcome was fairly predictable. They were choppy and awkward with such restrictions on their speech. They often tried to interrupt with "But . . ." statements. They were frustrated with me for staying so rigidly structured, even commenting that they thought I was supposed to be about respect! I grinned and admitted they were right and then begged them to continue the exercise. Once they had a chance to call me out on my tyrannical ways, they were more able to focus on what they were actually doing: listening to one another with more purpose and intent.

I then asked them how it felt to speak without interruption, how to be silent for that long, and then how it was to be able to affirm that they could hear one another and be heard pretty accurately. Grasping that they could better understand each other, if only a little, kept their interest in pursuing this path. We talked quite a bit about the value of being validated by the other, both agreeing that was what they both wanted more of in their relationship.

As time went on, they enhanced their abilities to listen more effectively but still ran into some significant blockades. Primary themes of conflict emerged. Whereas Will was struggling with his new identity as a gay man against his still-held traditional Christian beliefs and family values, Troy struggled equally with actually being in a committed relationship, especially to someone so new and unresolved to the gay lifestyle. But they both said repeatedly that they were very much in love and wanted to make this work.

So one day in the middle of a session, they were again discussing what a committed relationship looked like and meant to each of them. Will was saying that even if they couldn't get married legally, he wanted to have some kind of ceremony in a church. Troy, in total frustration said, "So what the hell is a little ceremony in a big church going to do? Is it going to fix your problems with being gay or feeling ashamed of going out with me to gay events?"

Will responded, "I hope that it does in time. I really want to feel more comfortable in my own skin and being out around others. And I definitely want to be out with you and your circle of friends. I'm not there yet, but I'm trying. The ceremony would help me because it would give me some blessing from God to move forward with my life, to feel forgiveness and to feel secure within myself again or maybe for the first time. Most of all, I want to tell the world how much I love you and try to make you feel more secure with me."

Troy was speechless for several minutes. He finally said, "I have never felt love before in my entire life. It scares me. I have never been loved by anyone before. It scares me even more. I feel safe and loved by you, which really, really scares the hell out of me because it's so damn hard to believe it could possibly last. I'm skeptical of your God because I've never had one and felt like if there were one, He or She would never approve of me. I'm still working on that. I love you more than I could ever imagine and also want to tell the world, but I feel hypocritical doing so in a church. Could we talk about other options?"
Will nodded yes, and the resulting embrace was long, sweet, and very tearful.

Several months later they planned a small ceremony out in a park with a minster and a handful of friends. They invited me, but I declined, citing my professional code of ethics. They showed me pictures later, and it was simply beautiful.

Less than a year later, gay marriage became legal, so they got married again with a justice of the peace and received all the legal benefits of marriage. Soon after, they adopted a child. They continued to check in with me periodically for several years. At our last check-in, they were planning a vacation with Will's biological son, Tony, and their adopted child, Cory, with the blessings of Will's former wife, who had forgiven Will for being who he really is and remains friends with him. Will and Troy report that they are truly happy as they grow more in validation and respect for one another.

Respect work with couples is complex because it means working intently with two individuals, helping them gain effective respect for themselves and each other, while at the same time, we are also addressing the functionality of the relationship they share. In both case studies, we can observe the conflicts of competitive needs to blame and shame one another can be respectfully redirected toward the issues of trust, forgiveness, and true intimacy, which intertwine to make a more enriched, caring relationship. Respect is primary to facilitate all three components in operating in a meaningful way.

In the next chapter, we will take the complexity of relationships and the individuals in them to yet a higher level. Families are networks of coexisting relationships within the system. We will take a closer look at those networks as well as all the persons who have simultaneous needs within that structure.

References

Bradley, B., & Furrow, J. L. (2004). Toward a mini-theory of the blamer softening event: Tracking the moment-by-moment process. *Journal of Marital and Family Therapy, 30*(2), 233–246.

Gottman, J., & Silver, N. (2012). *What makes love last?: How to build trust and avoid betrayal*. New York: Simon and Schuster.

Halling, S. (2008). *Intimacy, transcendence and psychology: Closeness and openness in everyday life*. New York: Palgrave-Macmillan.

Hendrick, S. S., Hendrick, C., & Logue, E. M. (2010). Respect and the family. *Journal of Family Theory & Review, 2*(2), 126–136.

Johnson, S. M., Hunsley, J., Greenberg, L., & Schindler, D. (1999). Emotionally focused couples therapy: Status and challenges. *Clinical Psychology: Science and Practice, 6*(1), 67–79.

Lawrence-Lightfoot, Sara. (2000). *Respect*. New York: Perseus Books.

Prager, K. J., & Roberts, L. J. (2004). Deep intimate connection: Self and intimacy in couple relationships. In *Handbook of closeness and intimacy*, Mashek, D.J., Aron, A., (Eds), Abingdon, England: Psychology Press, 43–60.

6   Parenting Respectfully

Helping Families Develop Healthy Bonds of Respect

Family therapy exponentially expands the process of untangling dysfunction from function and hurt from wholeness. In families there are more players and more dyads and triads to be understood as well as the individuals themselves. Respect within this system has many places to snag and often appears to be snagging everywhere.

In this chapter, much of the focus will be on parenting and the children in families because they are the most vulnerable. In many traditions, it has been long taught and assumed that children are to respect their elders unilaterally. RFT postulates that children need to be mutually honored, respected for who they are and are becoming, to learn how to better respect themselves and others around them.

Helping parents discover that children who experience genuine respect are more prepared to generate meaningful respect is key to RFT-oriented family therapy. With that understanding, parents frequently begin to explore their own inner child needs for respect and initiate a deeper understanding of respect for themselves as well. Therefore, we will concurrently explore how respect, or the lack thereof, impacts the entire system as well as each individual, dyad, and triad within that system.

As discussed in the previous chapter, Hendricks et al. (2010) highlight that respect is understudied as a construct generally in the social sciences but particularly so in family systems literature. They point specifically to the developmental nature of respect within the family: "Respect is complex and has many facets, including . . . developmental changes in respect awareness and action . . . the family is really the first 'small group' that an infant enters" (p. 131). The development is critical to understand. Respect is not inherent; it is learned through example and experience. Depending on not just what is taught but what is demonstrated and given directly to the child throughout the developmental years, respect for oneself and others can be nurtured effectively through parental (or other adult caretaker) modeling. Without the appropriate nurturance from a reliant and consistent source, it becomes more difficult for this critical piece of maturity to grow into genuine and healthy respect.

So if respect is experienced and learned in stages and if that process is interrupted by life events or the lack of familial respect, then it makes sense that those children, and the adults they become, are less vested in the notion of respect for themselves or others. This becomes generationally problematic in that parents continue to pass down lost respect or blatant disrespect to their children without intervention.

In family therapy, our first line of duty is to protect and thereby to respect the children in that family. This is not always a simple undertaking. We have a responsibility to assist the entire family. Indeed, the way to help children thrive within the family unit is to address the systemic needs of the family. Our objective is to decrease, if not eliminate, harm done by disrespectful patterns and help build more respectful interactions in each direction throughout the family unit. This means that all persons in that unit, big and small, will ultimately be able to give and receive respect with relative mutuality and equality in a caring and supportive way (Hendricks et al., 2010).

Because respect is a developmental learning experience, there is typically a disparity between the adult's capacity to render and manage this fuller kind of respect, which is greater than that of a child or adolescent. But often we see families in which this is not the case. The parents who come into therapy frequently have been so injured from their family of origin and prior generations that they are not able to adequately provide the level of respectful guidance the younger ones need.

Therefore, family therapists need to assess all of the dynamics at play. Too frequently, a child or adolescent is brought in and presented as "the problem," the one with attitudinal and behavioral problems, indicating that he or she has respect issues. This may be age appropriately valid, such as in adolescence, but it most often also reflects deeper conflicts within the family. Therefore, we need to explore what the obstructions to respect are in that young person's life, most significantly, those coming from the family.

Family Systems

A multitude of possible dyads and triads within the family make understanding the family system more complex. For example, the relationship between the parents may influence the relationships they independently have with each child and the triangulations that can occur as a result. The dyads and triads formed by siblings often reflect their parents' means of relating.

Bowen's Family Systems Theory (1993) indicates that there are dyadic conflicts, triangulations, power struggles, varied responses to traumas, losses, transitions, and so on as well as spoken or unspoken family rules and secrets. Depending on the severity of the dysfunction in a particular family, these layers may be distinct, or they may be blurred, overlapping in such a way that it is difficult to discern where and how all of the presenting pieces fit together.

In using the family systems approach with RFT, the work of the therapist includes assessing all conflicts, triangulations, power plays, trauma responses and rules and secrets in a way that offers genuine respect to each person as well as the family unit. In many families this can be a large undertaking because the strategies of the family have been embedded over several generations. The cumulative traumas can then become disempowering for the family such that the concept of mutual and equal respect becomes virtually nonexistent.

"Joining the family" is a concept shared by several family theorists, including Satir (1991)and Whitaker (1988). Both speak to the necessity of becoming actively engaged with the family to not appear as the detached observer but to be seen as one who joins in and is trusted to facilitate the family struggle toward change. Both put heavy emphasis on the therapist holding the belief and conviction that every family has the capacity for positive change and healing.

Whitaker (1988), from his Symbolic Experiential Approach, uses the metaphor of "being a coach of the entire baseball team rather than filling in for one position, say the first baseman" (p. 58). He further feels that it is absolutely necessary to have the entire team present to coach effectively. This means the entire family, both parents, all siblings, and as many extended family—aunts, uncles, cousins, grandparents, even boyfriends and girlfriends, and so on—as possible. Whereas this approach can be logistically untenable because many family members may be geographically spread apart, there is wisdom in being as all-inclusive as possible so as to not participate in splitting and further triangulating the members and being as inclusive of as many family members as possible.

Minuchen's (1974) Structural Family Therapy model addresses the family system by looking at how it functions as a whole, that is, how well the boundaries of that unit are working to allow a balance of autonomy and true connection within the family. The hierarchical structure of the family, as well as the subsystem dyads and triads, are "tracked" to understand the imbalances overall. The therapist using this model is asked to "join" the family so that she or he can assist in restructuring the various imbalanced places blocking growth and healing for everyone. The construct of respect once again emerges as the active agent for this restructuring process.

As we introduce, or reintroduce, the possibility of equalizing genuine respect for everyone within the family, we will probably be met with some opposition initially because we will be challenging the established strategies that are currently in place. We will address the triangulations and power plays by suggesting that those who are disenfranchised are also worthy of respect, particularly those who are children or adolescents.

However, this must be accomplished in ways that do not displace the respect for those who also need power and recognition. In other words, it is not enough to just advocate for the weakest; we must also engage the others in the experience of true respect, such that they too can appreciate what is being offered to everyone. In this manner, the more influential members can have a stake in creating a more respectful environment for everyone.

From a combined Family Systems and Attachment theory approach, the parents (or adult caregivers) also need to be securely attached to be able to create the same secure attachment for the child, as pointed out by Mikulincer, Florian, Cowan, and Cowan (2002): "The quality of parent-child relationships is the linking mechanism—that adults who are themselves securely attached tend to provide a secure base for their children" (p. 424). In other words, it is imperative to help parent figures gain their own sense of grounded respect and attachment, as much as possible, while also helping them create a stronger respectful bond with their child. This requires a delicate balance of paying attention to the available strengths as well as the relational needs for each parent and the ways in which these affect their interactions with their children.

The way in which a child responds to parents based on the historical pattern is quite significant. Additionally, what that child brings uniquely, that is, personality traits, resiliency, intelligence, special needs, and so on is an important factor in the developing dynamics of the family system (Crouter & Booth, 2003). So it is for each child in the family, not only in terms of relating to parent(s) but how that child interacts with siblings and others outside the home.

There are a multitude of possible influences on family dynamics, including those already mentioned as well as different configurations of modern families, such as single-parent households, blended families, extended family in the same household, and adoptive families. The endless number of possible family structural frameworks can create unique challenges to the therapeutic process. Learning ways to help the family deal with missing members through divorce, abandonment, illness, or death may be complicated by the triangulations formed in relation to that loss, that is, adult siblings triangulating after the death of a parent.

Figure 6.1 is a brief genogram showing how the RFT process is designed to work within a family.

Cultural differences such as race, nationality, religion, region, socioeconomics, and so on, which we will explore in greater depth in a later chapter, are equally significant and influential factors in the formation of family dynamics, as we will see in the following case study.

Relational Process With Families

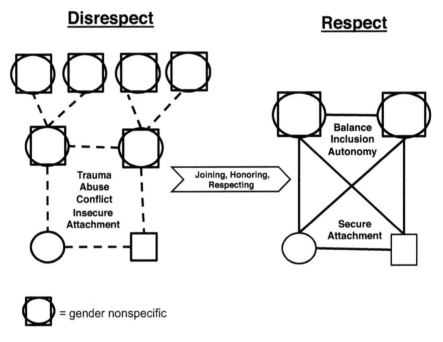

Figure 6.1 Relational Process With Families

Case in Point

Fred, a 56-year-old Hispanic man, and Angie, a 47-year-old African-American woman, brought their adolescent son, 14-year-old Marcus, into therapy because of behavioral issues at home, truancies from school, and suspected drug and gang activities.

Marcus has had a few brushes with police, mostly related to his truancies, trespassing, and loitering. He was accused of drug possession and dealing once, but no charges were made because of lack of evidence. He was held in juvenile detention for two nights, however, while that was decided. He claims that an officer threatened him with a gun and later hit him in the head with that same gun. No video was available to prove it. While he was in detention he met four older guys (15 and 16) who he described as "way cool," and they proceeded to induct him into their "gang," although Marcus insisted that it wasn't really a gang, just "a bunch of cool guys."

In their first family session, Fred explained that Marcus had attention deficit hyperactivity disorder (ADHD), that he had always had problems in school, and that he, Fred, understood this because he had had the same problem. In fact, Fred had done some prison time because he had a problem with drugs, although he said he was 3 years clean. The time in prison was for 5 years and ended 3 1/2 years ago.

Angie was more assertive in her body language and tone. She told me, in no uncertain terms, that, yes, her son was just like her husband, following in his footsteps. Tears appeared on her face as her tone got higher and louder. Pointing to Fred, she said, "He is a really bad influence on my children!" They had only one child in the room, Marcus, so I asked her to tell me more about the other children, partly to get more information about the family dynamics but also to deflect her accusatory attack on her husband.

She told me that there were five in total: two grown adults from her husband's previous marriage, Roberto, 28, and Tomas, 24. She also told me that she had a daughter, Laneisha, 21, out of wedlock. Together, they had two children, Marcus and his younger sister, Teana, age 12. Laneisha had been a bit of a "wild child," as Angie described her. "She's very smart, but she don't have much common sense!" she said, laughing. "All those trashy boys . . . I could have had as many boyfriends as my mom and Laneisha, but I didn't want them. Just too much trouble!" Teana, on the other hand, "is a good girl . . . very book smart. She likes school, studies a lot, stays out of trouble . . . kinda quiet like, you know?"

When I asked her more about Marcus, she just shook her head slowly. After a few minutes, she said softly, "To tell you the truth, Miss, I don't know what to think. He's my boy, and I love him a lot, but I'm scared. I'm scared that the way he's acting, he's either going to end up in jail, like his daddy and my daddy, or he's going to end up dead."

Marcus, who had been stoically quiet and aloof up until now, suddenly looked startled and scared. "No, I ain't," he almost screamed. Angie responded with, "Well, you know how the police treat Black men and boys!" With this, Marcus bowed, shaking his head, and withdrew from the conversation.

In this narrative about her children, she mentioned both of her parents, so I decided to ask more about her family of origin. A single mother raised Angie, although there were numerous boyfriends of her mother's in and out of their lives for as far back as Angie could remember. She had five siblings, one with the same father; the other four were half siblings. Angie was the oldest. She couldn't remember the last time she had seen her father. He was in jail for a little while and then, just after her younger brother was born, drifted off. She remembered most of the men in her life getting in some kind of trouble with the law, some because they deserved it but mostly because they were Black. She said that one of the reasons she'd married Fred was because he wasn't Black, and she thought she would be giving her children a better chance. "I really believed he'd be a better man and father," she said almost sarcastically.

Fred bit back harshly, "Your family is just a bunch of losers, and you know it!" And so it went for the rest of the session. Blame and shame flew across the room as Fred and Angie hurled their anger at one another. The identified client, Marcus, became invisible.

I soon realized that this was a well-worn pattern of triangulation within this family. The parents were focusing on the symptoms their child was exhibiting as the problem to be solved in therapy—the "fix my kid" syndrome versus looking at what is going on behind the scenes, namely the dyadic problems between Fred and Angie, which in turn, set up the triangulation problems with Marcus. He is being put in the middle of their conflict, which he cannot and should not have to manage. He really has only two options: to divert attention away from the conflict through his acting out or to withdraw as completely as possible from the conflict, becoming invisible. With this in mind and the concern I was beginning to have for Marcus being further scapegoated, I invited in his siblings for our next session.

To my surprise, all the siblings, Roberto, Tomas, Laneisha, and Teana accompanied Marcus and parents to the next session. In the beginning it was mayhem. There were eight people in my office, myself included. We had to bring in three extra chairs from the waiting room, which fit snugly around the perimeter of the room. The two older brothers took the extra chairs nearest the door. Fred and Angie sat on the sofa with Teana joining them; Laneisha grabbed the chair nearest me but also nearest the window, leaving the last side chair beside the sofa for Marcus. All the men, including Marcus, were large in build, so the room felt even tighter and a bit stuffy. I asked if everyone was comfortable and adjusted the air-conditioning accordingly.

After introducing myself to the new members and greeting and thanking each one individually for coming, I offered my summary of what I understood the goals for family therapy in general to be, namely to help everyone in the family to have a voice in the process and to facilitate conflict resolutions necessary for better family unity. I asked if that met with their expectations. Initially everyone nodded passively, but then, Roberto spoke up, saying, "Wait a minute, I thought we were here to help Marcus get his shit together!"

Tomas and Laneisha quickly chimed in, agreeing completely with Roberto. They were told by their parents that they were there to help fix Marcus. Laneisha let it be known that she thought this was "a complete waste of time because only Marcus could fix his problems and other people had bigger problems anyway."

At this point Angie spoke up, "Everybody, give the counselor a chance." And then to me she said, "Look, Miss, the real truth is that we probably all need your help. But right now we're really worried about Marcus 'cause he's going down the wrong path, just like his father and them two boys," while pointing to Roberto and Tomas.

Their reactions were to be expected. They both immediately stood up and started to leave. I interjected that I understood that they were angry, but asked if they would please reconsider and stay for a few more minutes. They stalled for a minute or two, muttering under their breaths, but did eventually sit back down. Fred leered at Angie and sharply said, "You have no right to talk to my two boys that way!"

Angie started to respond vigorously, but I stopped her by gently tapping her arm. I thanked her for helping me better understanding the problem as she saw it. I quickly followed up by saying that I appreciated everyone in the room for being courageous enough to be here in my small office with one another despite the discomfort it may cause. I voiced my recognition that there were different points of view in the room as well as an assortment of different feelings, including some unpleasant ones, including anger. Everyone unanimously agreed with that! I smiled and noted that we had our first group agreement. A few chuckles followed. I affirmed that it was more than OK to disagree and that each person in the room had equal rights to their perspectives, opinions, and feelings. The hard part for everyone was knowing how to deal with those thoughts and feelings when they conflicted with others, especially the people we care most about. Silence accompanied people looking down at their shoes, which was the only response.

I then shifted my focus to Marcus and his younger sister, Teana. I asked them both how they were feeling about being here at this point, and they both shrugged. I said to Marcus that it must be really hard being the star attraction here. He grinned at me and said, "Yes ma'am, it really is!" I asked him what the hardest part about all of this was for him so far. He put his face in his hands and appeared to be thinking about that intensely. Others became restless and agitated, while he thought, but I motioned for quiet patience, please. He finally answered in a low voice, "I think that they're all mad at me because I'm acting like them." I asked him to explain whom he meant by "they," and he motioned toward his dad and older half-brothers.

After a minute or two, I asked about his mom, "Is she angry too . . . for the same reason?"

He looked at her and shook his head. "She's just scared I'm going to turn out like them—go to jail and stuff."

"Are you scared too?"

"No! . . . I don't know. . . . It don't really matter."

I responded with "It really does matter," *looking in his eyes. We ended the session soon after that. I invited everyone to come back but got nonverbal feedback indicating that the older siblings had no such plans.*

My case notes from this session stated the following: that parents were divided by their expectations of one another, showing insecure attachment styles that probably reflected the patterns learned in their families of origin. The children of each parent were divided accordingly, triangulating against the stepparents and the two they had together, who were caught in the middle. Teana, being younger and female, seemed less torn, more closely aligned with her mother, but also with her brother, Marcus was the one most conflicted and thereby scapegoated. I planned to start the next session asking Teana about what mattered most in the family as well as for her.

When we next met, I began by asking for a check-in from all the family members in the room, as I always do. As predicted, only Fred, Angie, Marcus, and Teana were there. Initially, no one had much to say. Headshakes, shrugs, and quiet "I'm fine(s)" *went around the room as I looked at each person. After a pause, I looked at Teana and asked if she could help me out for a few minutes. With a quizzical look, she said,* "Sure."

I explained to her that what I'd like to learn was her perspective on what was going on within her family. What did she think caused the most conflict at home? She answered that it was Marcus always getting into trouble. I asked her why he was always getting in trouble. She shrugged but then said she guessed it was to get attention, which Marcus immediately denied. I then asked her why she thought Marcus needed to seek attention. She eventually replied that maybe it was because he was tired of hearing Mom and Dad fighting all the time. I asked her if she was tired of it too, and she vigorously shook her head yes. I thanked her for helping me out.

Meanwhile, Marcus was fuming. I asked him what was wrong. He almost shouted, "I don't seek no attention. I just seem to always get it, if I want it or not!" *Angie spoke up,* "Well, why do you keep getting in trouble then?" *Marcus sighed heavily and shut down.*

Fred had his head down, looking at his lap, and whispered to Angie, "Leave the boy the God-damn alone!" *I asked Fred how he was feeling.*

He yelled, "I'm pissed . . . pissed at her for always being so high and mighty! She always thinks she's so good—better than everyone else!" Angie's response was that she had never gone to jail and was just trying to teach her children right from wrong. This led into a shouting match between Fred and Angie over who was the better parent. It was finally halted by an unexpected scream from Marcus, who ordered, "Shut the hell up!" Everyone froze. Here was a perfect opportunity to open a discussion around respect, but I decided to save it for the next session and terminated this one 10 minutes early.

At this point in therapy, the chaos in the family was really beginning to reveal itself. It was obvious that respect was not functionally present in any direction because no individual had enough to hold onto, much less to share. Fred had a deep load of internal shame from his past, which Angie reinforced through her resentment and humiliation from the disappointments and abuses she had experienced from the men in her past. The generational depletion of respect had left this family void of the experiential awareness of what true respect looks or feels like. The parents were scrambling to gather any fragments of respect they could find for themselves without really being able to identify what that meant, while each of the children were equally mystified, yet just as hungry for it. Out of this collective hunger came the desire to strike out or to retreat. The job ahead was to introduce the concept of respect in such a way that it felt more tangible and attainable for every member of the family to achieve equitably.

For Marcus to be able to yell "Shut the hell up!" to his parents was empowering and liberating for him, yet not helpful in terms of learning about the value of respect for himself or others. I had to help him take that experience in a different direction.

So, in opening the next session, I started by processing with everyone what the last few minutes of the last session had felt like to each of them. After a few moments, Angie just shook her head and said it didn't feel good to her at all. "That was very disrespectful, very, very disrespectful!" Fred nodded in agreement. Marcus just grinned.

Teana finally spoke up, "I was scared." The grin on Marcus's face disappeared, and he quickly asked why, with some fear of his own. She told him that it seemed like a big, scary crash in their family that never went away. "All the arguing and anger just keeps happening. I'm just scared to do or say anything!" As her eyes watered, so did his and then Angie's. "I just want this all to stop," Teana said.

After a significant pause, I asked each person in the room to think about what it might look and feel like for the arguing and anger to stop. Everyone agreed that it would be good, but no one had any ideas about how to make it happen. Fred finally spoke up. "I've been *angry my whole life. My daddy was angry and mean when he drank, and so was his daddy. I grew up scared of when I was going to get my next beating or when my mama was. I never knew there was anything different. So I guess I did the same thing outta self-protection, I guess. I'm not sure I can ever change after so many years."*

After a longer pause, I asked the others if they thought anything could change and what that might take. No one was sure, but they thought they would have to be nicer to each other.

Weeks went by as we continued to talk about what respect in the family might be like and how we could help it grow. There were still fights happening, some severe, especially when Marcus got suspended from school again. He had gotten into a fight with another kid, who he said started the fight. After some bickering in the family about whose fault it was, I asked Marcus if he knew of any way he could have stopped or prevented the scuffle. He said no, but Teana said, "You could have respected yourself enough to walk away." Fred started to object, to say that real men don't do that, but after a loving look from Angie—something I had not seen before—Fred changed his demeanor and said, "It takes a lot of courage . . . but sometimes it's just the right thing to do." Angie squeezed his arm and whispered, "Thank you." I summarized the session by acknowledging the efforts taken by everyone to be more thoughtful and appreciative of each other by stopping and thinking about how to approach problems differently.

It turned out that Fred and Angie had been talking more openly during the weeks that we had been addressing the issue of respect in the family. This was critical to the healing and restructuring of the family. All of the patterns of triangulations, scapegoating, blaming, and shaming were still there, but they all were melting slowly as the distrust and resentments in the parents' relationship began to heal. Much work was ahead of us, but the healing process had begun.

I decided to invite just the couple to come in for a few sessions. I explored with them what changes, if any, they were beginning to notice in the family. They shrugged at first but did say that the two of them were starting to feel better. No, they didn't know why exactly. There was still a good amount of conflict in the house, which the older kids from both sides were passive-aggressively feeding into, and Marcus's behavior was a little better but still troubling. But at least they were talking more.

They told me about a discussion they had had between the two of them a couple of days prior to this appointment. Angie had been irritated with Fred all day because he had been watching TV and playing video games nonstop for the better part of 2 days. Meanwhile Angie said she had gone to work, washed dishes, and prepared dinner. She *had finally had enough and told Fred so. A hot argument ensued until Fred said, "Stop!" He reminded Angie as well as himself that they needed to be more respectful toward one another and then apologized to her for not helping more. He explained that he had been working double shifts lately, was tired, and did not feel well, but knew that wasn't a good excuse. Angie, ready to fire back, was stunned by his apology. She started to cry, saying that she couldn't remember when anyone had apologized to her so directly.*

They continued to talk for 2 more hours that night. Angie opened up regarding her deep hurts and disappointments with her mother and all the men who paraded in and out of their lives. Some of them had been really mean to her if not outright abusive. Her trust in men had been shattered completely.

In turn Fred shared how he had been so completely shattered by his father's wrath. He came from a long line of alcoholics and knew it. He swore to himself as a child that he would never turn out like them, and then he did. He became very depressed in jail, feeling like a complete failure. He even felt like committing suicide at one point but knew he couldn't do that to his family. He apologized again to Angie for not being a better husband and father but said that he really did love her and wanted to do better.

This open emotional conversation was pivotal to the progress to be made with the rest of the family. It would take months and beyond for all of the members to learn how to interact in a healthier manner, but the road was now less blocked.

As Angie and Fred became familiar with using more respectful language toward one another and themselves, they also learned how to use it more effectively with their children. They became less critical of Marcus. In fact, they learned to recognize and compliment him on his merits. For example, when he completed summer school and was then able to advance to the next grade, Fred and Angie took him out to dinner and told him how proud they were of him.

That next school year was a little bumpy in the beginning for Marcus, but he was able to turn it around soon enough to start making better grades. He even let it slip in one of our last sessions that he actually liked history and math, which I teased him about, saying that I had that on tape! As he built more self-respect and confidence, he started choosing different friends, and reduced his gang-like behaviors dramatically.

Before terminating with this family, I invited all of the half-siblings to join in a complete family session. Pleasantly surprised, I noted that they all came back. Silence began the session, but I also noted far less tension in the room. Tomas and Laneisha were actually smiling. I mentioned that it felt lighter in the room than it had before. Laneisha spoke up first, saying that she and her mom were on much better speaking terms now than they had been in years. Tomas chimed in, saying, yea, he and his dad were tighter than he could remember, and Roberto nodded in agreement. I asked Fred, Angie, and the other two kids what they thought about this, and they all agreed that things had been much better lately.

Toward the end of the session, Teana spoke up, "I feel like I have a much bigger and better family now. I even like Roberto more, except when he gets on my nerves, teasing me about my boyfriend!" They both laughed.

References

Bowen, M. (1993). *Family therapy in clinical practice.* New York: Jason Aronson.

Crouter, A. C., & Booth, A. (Eds.). (2003). *Children's influence on family dynamics: The neglected side of family relationships.* New York: Routledge.

Hendrick, S. S., Hendrick, C., & Logue, E. M. (2010). Respect and the family. *Journal of Family Theory & Review,* 2(2), 126–136. c5, 6.

Mikulincer, M., Florian, V., Cowan, P. A., & Cowan, C. P. (2002). Attachment security in couple relationships: A systemic model and its implications for family dynamics. *Family Process,* 41(3), 405–443.

Minuchin, S. (1974). *Families and family therapy.* Cambridge, MA: Harvard University Press.

Satir, V., & Banmen, J. (1991). *The Satir model: Family therapy and beyond.* Mountain View, CA: Science & Behavior Books.

Whitaker, C., & Bumberry, W. M. (1988). *Dancing with the family.* New York: Brunner/Mazel.

7 Group Therapy
Strangers Learning to Respect Themselves and Others

Group therapy has many beneficial components, which serve well to be enhanced by the concepts of RFT. To begin, it is usually made up of individuals who have no history with one another. Therefore, there is a "clean slate" of relational patterns among them. They bring with them their own personal and relational woundedness, but they are now in a fresh environment that offers an opportunity for shifts in self-evaluations as well as perceptions of others, which can result in change in a more respectful understanding and interaction. This change, hopefully, will transition into a broader awareness of respect for humanity in a larger transpersonal framework.

Looking deeper into the process and dynamics of group therapy, we find more avenues for RFT to be instrumental in setting the groundwork for growth and change. In the development of group cohesion, new rules for interactive engagement are formed. Because there is no historical pattern to be followed, the discovery of respect for self and others is more attainable.

So it is the job of therapists to move this group of strangers into connection with one another in a new way of bonding. Their individual styles of relating will emerge in ways that initially look like conflict, typically heightened by the insecure nature of strangers meeting strangers. Helping each person move past that sense of insecurity into some sense of comfort and belonging is key to further support and cohesion within the group. Using RFT, the therapist offers the first stage of respect by genuinely welcoming each person into the group and demonstrating ways of showing true respect for every person in the room, equally and fairly. This will set the crucial stage for creating the framework on which the dynamic of respect can develop.

Creating and maintaining the precedent of respectful relating will often prove to be challenging because the unrelated participants bring in their anxieties about the safety of a new group experience as well as the pain from their past and the maladaptive patterns those pains have manifested prior to the group experience.

Group Process

With these factors in mind, the nature of group process and related dynamics need to be carefully considered. As Corey, Corey, and Corey (2013) suggest:

> Group process . . . includes dynamics such as the norms that govern a group, the level of cohesion in the group, how trust is generated, how resistance is manifested, how conflict emerges and is dealt with, forces that bring about healing, inter-member reactions, and the various stages in a group's development. (p. 5)

It is in these stages that group therapy can be truly dynamic, allowing the momentum for positive, respectful change.

Yalom and Leszcz (2008) list 11 primary factors necessary in the group process:

1 Instillation of hope
2 Universality
3 Imparting information
4 Altruism
5 The corrective recapitulation of the primary family group
6 Development of socializing techniques
7 Imitative behavior
8 Interpersonal learning
9 Group cohesiveness
10 Catharsis
11 Existential factors (p. 1)

Of these, four factors stand out in terms of relating more specifically to the tenets of RFT: the instillation of hope, universality, altruism, and interpersonal learning. The instillation of hope refers to inherently setting the belief in the client's ability to grow and change in a positive way, thus allowing the client to hold onto that belief as well. This expands easily into the RFT notion that each person deserves the recognition of strengths and the ability to move beyond current life circumstances.

Yalom further addresses the client's sense of alienation and stranger anxiety with the concept of universality. That is, each member who joins a group brings some fear that his or her own unique secrets of shame might be revealed to this group of strangers in a more humiliating and harmful way. The shared human experience of feeling inadequate or shameful becomes evident as stories are told, and the realization of this universal truth then can powerfully provide some comfort and relief that each person is not isolated but part of humanity. Within this discussion of universality, Yalom also addresses the complexities of multiculturalism and the therapeutic need to be aware and sensitive to the particular sociocultural differences there might be in the group and the power disparities that these may cause. More will be discussed regarding multiculturalism later in this chapter and in the next.

Altruism and interpersonal learning both speak to the process of gaining respect for others. Yalom's discourse on interpersonal learning lends itself to attachment theory by suggesting that we all need a sense of belonging and emotional nurturance beginning from early childhood. When that attachment, or sense of belonging, breaks down or never existed, then "relational distortions" emerge. Therefore, Yalom posits that all mental health issues rest in, and are corrected by, more interpersonal and emotional exchanges that move from the negative to the more positive. Respect, then, is the shift needed and hopefully supplied in a group therapy setting. Yalom argues that everyone needs to feel needed, and when one can give to another unselfishly, then one profits by that act also. The emotional correction comes from the awareness that "I" have positive value in relating to others.

What the RFT therapist brings to this table for discussion is the continued primary focus on increasing the amount of respectful energy in the room: the therapist both fully respects where each person in the group is concurrently, including the resistance that comes naturally in the process, and fosters discovery of respect for each client. These parallel functions open the door to the client's new awareness and experience, which enables him or her to work out internal and interpersonal conflicts.

For the rest of this chapter we will be looking closer at the dynamics of group therapy and how those dynamics can be strengthened and supported by RFT (see Figure 7.1). We will begin by looking into the ways in which individuals in the group can develop greater self-compassion and

Group Therapy Process

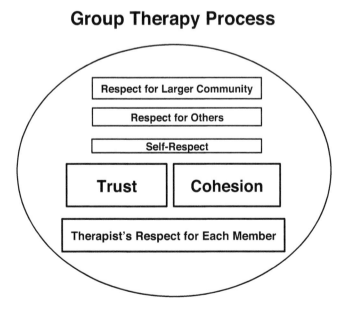

Figure 7.1 Group Therapy Process

respect for oneself, followed by how those in a group can master greater respect for others through thoughtful intention, discussion, and action, doing or saying respectful things toward others. Finally, we will consider ways in which group work might serve to expand upon those dynamics to include more universal understandings, those which are more socially inclusive and accepting. This may seem to be a rather large bridge to cross, but the process of gaining greater respect outside of our previous experiences leads to a prospect of gaining a larger appreciation for persons of different perspectives, beliefs, societies, and cultures as well as our own.

Self-Respect and Compassion Building in Groups

One of the key components or goals of any group process is to encourage and render the outcome of improved self-regard for each member of the group. The regard for oneself can be understood through a slightly different lens, compassion, and still achieve similar results. Self-compassion, as studied by Gilbert and Procter (2006) in their research demonstrating the effectiveness of "Compassionate Mind Training," offers the client the opportunity to reexamine his or her pattern of shame and self-criticism in a more constructive way. In this study, they offered a 12-week therapy group in an inpatient setting to deeply self-critical patients. They implemented the Compassionate Mind Training process. The theory behind the process considers shame and subsequent self-criticism to be major negative contributors to many different forms of mental illness diagnoses, most notably, depression and anxiety. They cite support for such a claim from several perspectives, such as attachment theory and Dialectical Behavior Therapy.

These authors view shame and self-criticism as very destructive elements to one's mental health and, therefore, are the targeted components to be changed by compassion and warmth for oneself. That is, these thoughts, feelings, beliefs, and actions considered by the researchers to be most dangerous were explained to the clients as being protective strategies that they learned to use to combat fear or vulnerability. By framing those very harmful elements in a nonconfrontational way to the patients, they offered compassion to the problem so that the patient could also address it compassionately. With receiving direct feedback from the patients themselves and their own observations, a substantial drop in shame and self-criticism was noted.

Likewise, RFT aims for similar results by replacing disrespect for oneself with a greater sense of grounded respect, building a sense of internal care and concern with the support of the group. The differences between compassion and respect may seem minimal but worth considering. Compassion refers to warmth, feeling, and empathy, whereas respect contains empathy plus a more cognitive sense of value and worth.

Respect for Others Through Intention and Practice

Respecting others is an equally important goal in RFT group work. Paré, Bondy, and Malhotra (2006) address this issue of learning how to respect others in a uniquely direct way. They present their work with groups of men who are in treatment for abusing their partners. Critical to their primary objective in therapy are the differences in talking about the *intention* of respect versus *performing* respect. Whereas they note that dialog is a form of "doing" and encourage the narrative of intention, they emphasize the need for *enactments* or role plays of actual situations with partners in which they find barriers to actually behaving or speaking in respectful and nonviolent ways to their partners. Some of these barriers include cultural belief systems like "men should never back down or apologize" or personal experiences of witnessing or being abused.

The researchers emphasize that they work toward "externalizing" or separating the person from the problem. The purpose of this externalization is to help the person not overidentify with the problem behavior, manifesting paralyzing shame that disengages positive change, but rather to approach the destructive patterns more objectively. By watching an enactment that reflects his inability to act respectfully, the way he intends, he is more able to conceptualize the interchange differently and modify his means of relating with the interactive support from the group.

This particular model clearly demonstrates the full purpose of RFT. Performing respect is more than a step beyond just talking about it. In fact, it is the primary goal to move respectful rapport and dialog into active engagement in the client's daily life. This assimilation process is the therapeutic outcome, which not only affords empowerment but also provides a smoother on-ramp to stronger social and personal relationships. Through modeling and active discussion in the room about the meaning, purpose, and the intention of respect, as well as the experiential benefits, ground is prepared for active respectful performance.

This action cannot be forced but allows greater access through unblocking the existing barriers, as Pare et al. (2006) suggest. These barriers encompass the fears that get in the way of trust and intimacy and the restrictive anger that dominates over all other emotions that suggest vulnerability. Helping clients gain safety around experiencing the softer emotions for themselves often allows that same safety to broaden toward others. In other words, allowing the walls of disrespect to come down provides room for a different dynamic to grow in an active dimension, that of behaving more respectfully.

Multiculturalism

Groups are normally formed with perfect strangers who have some specific struggles in common, be it anxiety, depression, anger, abuse, and so on. The group process is designed to bring them together so that they can collectively work on those common struggles. However, their "stranger-ness," or lack of connection outside of the group, sets up a unique phenomenon. Each of the individuals in that selected group is confronted with not only different personalities and personal circumstances, but they have to also deal with a variety of familial and cultural backgrounds. They have no shared history. This presents a different challenge for the RFT group therapist.

Respect then becomes larger in scope. It becomes a challenging exercise that reaches beyond oneself or known others; it becomes universal or transpersonal. Accordingly, Green and Stiers (2002) discuss multiculturalism that exists within the group dynamic and process. They point out that in addition to the therapeutic process designed to address various psychological issues, there is concurrently a social construct to be recognized and addressed. They speak of multiculturalism as "the inclusion in our therapeutic dialogues of the broad range of significant differences (race, gender, sexual orientation, ability and disability, religion, class, etc.) that often hinders communication and understanding" (p. 234). Without the full recognition of these social differences, we stay unaware of the power and privilege disparities that exist among the group.

Case in Point

A few years ago I led an outpatient adolescent girls group that focused primarily on body image, sexuality, and self-esteem. The group ran for 8 weeks. The topics for discussion revolved around self and body image, relationships, and sexuality as they relate to trauma. There were five members, as listed and described.

Melanie, Caucasian, 15 years old, came from a low-income family who lived in a trailer on the outskirts of town. She had two siblings, both younger than her. Her parents had been divorced for 3 years. Mom, a meth user, took off with another man 2 weeks before the divorce was final. Melanie and her siblings were living with Dad, who was an alcoholic, going in and out of periods of sobriety and rarely home. He had a history of depression and physical abuse toward Melanie's mother. Melanie ran away often, was on probation for truancy and pot possession, was a cutter, and had been hospitalized twice for suicidal ideation.

Cindy, Vietnamese, 14 years old, was American born but lived in a community and family who spoke predominately Vietnamese and was isolated, for the majority, from Westerners. Cindy's maternal grandparents fled from Vietnam during the war but never learned English. They ran a small grocery store, serving mostly Vietnamese, which her parents took over when the grandparents retired. Cindy, an only child, had had great difficulty assimilating into her middle school, as she also had a cleft palette, and had been bullied harshly by several gang members, one of whom also tried to rape her unsuccessfully. She, too, battled with depression and some suicidal thoughts.

Andrea, African-American, 16 years old, lived with her auntie, two brothers who were both older than she, and four cousins, all younger. She grew up with a young single mother, never knowing her father as he was in prison, presumably falsely arrested for theft. Mother had had several boyfriends since, one of whom introduced Andrea's mom to heroin and molested Andrea. Several years ago CPS stepped in and removed Mother's parental rights, placing guardianship with her sister, Auntie Carol, who held a stable job and proved to be a good, nurturing parent. Andrea very proudly and defiantly stated that she had no problems, got good grades in school, and planned on going to college. But she also got very angry, very quickly, and had been suspended from school several times for getting into fights with teachers and other students.

Lucia, Hispanic, 14, had lived in the US for 4 years. She understood English but had difficulty speaking it. She came here with her older sister Maria, 19, who was now going to college. They came looking for their father, who had moved to the US years ago, and they had not heard from him since. Unfortunately, they found out he had died soon after he had gotten here in a scuffle with the police, as they were trying to round up "illegal aliens." Their father actually had a work visa but wasn't given the time to prove it.

Their mother was still in Mexico, too ill to travel. Lucia has been tested to have some learning disabilities and was 3 months pregnant. She has missed a lot of school.

Pam, 17, Muslim, from New York originally, said she hated Texas and all Southerners. Pam's parents divorced 2 years ago, right before her mother moved to Texas with Pam and her two younger siblings to be with her mother's sister. Her father was Palestinian and still lived in New York, living with his girlfriend, his mistress before the divorce. Pam reported that he was verbally, emotionally, and physically abusive toward her mother, but that she, Pam, had a very good relationship with her father and missed him very much. Pam had struggled with bulimia in the past but had recently completed treatment for eating disorders and claimed to be symptom free and in recovery.

In the initial session, I began the group with a robust welcome, inviting each member to introduce and tell a little about themselves, acknowledging their presence with direct eye contact and a big smile. Afterward I commented about each person's unique story and perspective. I followed by saying that I was also aware of some commonalities among them, such as the experience of pain, but also the will to survive and improve their lives in meaningful ways. In so doing, I set the stage for more hopeful, respectful interaction to be possible.

However, the group got off to rocky start because of rivalry among three of the girls: Melanie, Andrea, and Pam. It quickly became apparent that each of these three girls needed and aggressively sought primary attention. The other two, Cindy and Lucia, were much more passive, presumably because of the language barriers, but they stayed engaged with the conversation, be it quietly. Andrea and Pam were the first to head into conflict. They struggled for domination of the group by both getting louder early in the group process, attempting to establish who had a worse home life. As they fought, Melanie joined in stating that no one could possibly have a worse childhood and present circumstances than she. As she began to cry, tears started rolling down the faces of Lucia and Cindy as well. Cindy hid her face as she was ashamed of the tears.

As this went into the second session, voices got louder as the three campaigned for who had the most misery. I stepped in by suggesting that it sounded like each of the three had a great deal of pain to talk about, as did the other two who had not yet spoken. I then reflected back each of the three personal stories shared thus far, offering respect for their pain and the persons they each were. I also asked if there were other stories to share, getting affirmative facial expressions from the other two but no verbal responses just yet.

Over the next couple of sessions we talked more about the personal stories shared. Pam and Andrea continued to seek the majority of attention, so I directed their storytelling in a way that common themes or feelings could be recognized. For example, when Pam talked about how angry she was that her parents divorced and she was now so far from her father, I suggested that might be similar to the way Andrea and Lucia felt by not having their fathers around either. The more the connection of life experiences was made clearer, the softer the tone became.

More attention was purposely focused on the others, trying to provide more balanced connection in the group. The language barriers for both Cindy and Lucia proved to be a challenge to ensure that they each had the chance to process what was being said and that they were each permitted ample time and space to speak. This was not well received by the dominant ones at first, but it did open a small window to let the quieter voices be heard.

Thoughtful silence also needed to be established for everyone to attend to the inner voices in the group. This required patience from me, as a therapist, to create the space for respectful reflection to be available to each of the members. Silence can prove to be uncomfortable to many, especially adolescents, and is typically filled with nervous giggles and stares. This was not an exception here, although agitation grew quickly from there. I remained calm but vigilant about reminding everyone during these times to breathe deeply and listen carefully to her inner voice. What were they feeling inside, and how did they want to respond to those feelings? We practiced some mindfulness by paying attention to how and where in their bodies they were feeling stress and how to respond to that stress with relaxation. This undoubtedly took some time but slowly reduced the tension in the group significantly.

In our fourth session, Pam was unusually quiet. When she did finally speak, she spoke softly. She hadn't heard from her father for 3 weeks, and she didn't want to admit that he might be pulling away from her, although that was what she most dreaded. So she sat awkwardly silent, fidgeting in her chair. Andrea asked her if she had tried to contact him, with no response. Melanie started to speak to Pam and got an immediate evil eye in return. She retreated for a minute but then did say, "I live with my dad, and I still miss him. He's hardly ever home, and when he is, he's usually drunk."

After a few moments, Lucia's head straightened up to speak. She said slowly, softly, and deliberately, "I miss my papa too." Everyone turned and really looked at her for the first time. I asked her to explain what that was like for her. At first, she bowed her head, saying she didn't know. Then she said in deliberate but broken English, "My father was my hero. He came to this country to give my family a better life, and he got killed for it. I don't understand why anybody would do a thing like that. He was a good man and worked hard always. . . . I thought the father of my baby was just like him, but he was a coward. He was too afraid of his responsibilities. He ran away as soon as I told him I was pregnant and wouldn't get an abortion."

Andrea spoke up and said she did know, even if she never met her father, and it was awful. I was beginning to fear that this was turning into another one-upmanship, when Cindy spoke up and said, "I've not lost my father, and I can't imagine what that would be like. Terrible, I guess. I think it would be different for everyone and yet kind of the same."

She went on, "My mother and father are very kind people but very timid. Their parents were also very timid because they were treated brutally after the war. I am also timid because of them and because my speech and knowledge of English is not good. The kids at school tease me and bully me a lot because I'm different. I ask my parents for help, but they don't know how. Some of the kids bully me so much;

they try to hurt me (tears) . . . They try to rape me. Only, I'm not that kind of girl! They think I'm a bad girl, but I'm not. I'm just weak (more tears)."

The other girls, who I was pretty certain had never encountered a person with a cleft palette before, had not engaged with her by eye contact or conversation before. They showed visible signs of being uncomfortable. There was a long silence. I suggested that it did not seem like weakness at all to me to be in a new place and be in a vulnerable space to encounter bullying. In fact, it takes strength to be there at all. The bullies are the weak ones because they are the ones who don't honor themselves, much less human differences in others.

Several girls started to squirm. Then, Lucia spoke up. "I too have been bullied. I didn't know the right word for that, so thank you. But that is really why I got pregnant. I was so lonely and so sad when I found out my father was dead. I just needed somebody to talk to. This kid, this guy, my baby's father, said he would take care of me. He fed me, let me stay with him and his father when my sister and I fought, spoke Spanish with me, but then he made me have sex with him. My sister doesn't believe me, but I swear it's true. I didn't love him—I hate him now because he left me on my own, and my sister doesn't want to help me either." She had a decision to make about her baby, to keep it or not, and she didn't know what to do, especially with no support. I told her that I would speak to her privately about what resources were available but that it was ultimately a decision only she and her sister could make.

The others acknowledged the difficult position she was in and then noted the similar circumstances Cindy was in as well. They talked for a while about the problems of bullying at school and that they all had experienced it at one time or another.

I spoke to the group about their shared bravery in relating such personal pain. Talking about such private thoughts and feelings took courage and real inner strength. I thanked them all for trusting each other and me enough to be vulnerable and real in this group.

As the next session progressed, the girls talked about the more current events in their lives, school, boys, friends, their favorite music, and so on, a common response to becoming so vulnerable in a group setting before true cohesion is fully developed. Sprinkled into the conversation were comments about how they felt about their moms and themselves.

For instance, when Melanie spoke about her best friend at school, saying, "And she has the best mom ever! My mom never took me shopping or anything. She said she didn't have time to do stuff with me. And then she just took off." Or when Cindy talked about not having any friends at school, she said, "I don't know how to make friends at school. My mother doesn't have any friends either. She's too scared to try, and so am I." Andrea said bluntly, "I don't have a mother. She loves her drugs and her men more than me, and I don't think she loves them or herself very much either." Andrea immediately jumped from that statement to declaring how much she hated her math teacher because she always talks down to her, trying to make her feel dumb, so Andrea has to yell at her to prove how smart she really is.

In our following session, I opened the group with our usual check-in from the previous week, only I added one request. I asked them to think about saying one or two words about how they were feeling about themselves this week. Initially, the response were cookie-cutter "fine" and "good," but Lucia, who was third to speak, said, "I feel ashamed. Girls at school called me a Mexican whore! Maybe I am. Am I?" After a few seconds, Andrea spoke up, "No. I lived with a whore all my life, so I should know. I'm the stereotypic Black girl who grew up without a dad and had a whore for a mother. What does that make me?" Tears started rolling down on both of these girls' faces.

The other three looked on with a sense of fear and panic. They didn't know what to say. I suspected that a good part of that panic was also about their own sense of shame, which sat deeply inside of all of them. I then said, "I believe that we all carry some shame because no one is perfect. Life experiences can and often do block our abilities to see the beauty and goodness that is also in us. But it really is there. We just have to cut the weeds down enough that we can see it."

A few eyes rolled along with some smiles, but Melanie shook her head violently, saying, while sobbing, "Nothing can cut down my weeds!" There was dead silence in the room for several minutes. I sat in silence with them, acknowledging the enormity of their pain.

At this point in the group process I was aware that a deeper trust and bond was developing slowly because they were each sharing their stories in a less competitive, more open way. The girls were struggling collectively to find a means of honoring themselves in their trauma-burdened lives. Therefore, they were ill equipped to sufficiently honor or support one another. Instead it seemed that one person's trauma only triggered another's. A shift needed to take place in the dynamic of this group, one that would allow for greater awareness of personal value that stood apart from the devaluing events in each of their lives.

As the weeks went on, we talked more about honoring their pain with compassion but also how to begin honoring themselves as human beings of worth and value in spite of the pain. We discussed the meaning of dignity and how they could claim it for themselves. Important to the discussion was the concept of separating our identity from the identity of others. This meant not internalizing the shame of others or the shame others try to place on us. To this point, I asked each of them to think about a different statement they could say at the end of each of the sessions that would clearly own their unique value and strengths. Here are some of the responses from this exercise after several weeks of practicing:

> *Melanie: I deserve to live a good life. I can cut down my own weeds.*
> *Cindy: I can and do belong here or anywhere.*
> *Lucia: My life matters and so does the life of my baby.*
> *Andrea: I am smart enough to make good choices.*
> *Pam: I am loved always because I love myself.*

As they began to genuinely internalize these messages that they were giving to themselves, they had a larger capacity to hear others' stories from a stronger place, such that they could listen more compassionately without being as triggered. I then asked them to say something affirming about the worthiness of one another. As they did so, they each found a new dimension for themselves; they became more nurturing and respectful of one another. I gave my reflections on the personal growth that I had seen in each girl and asked them to do the same. As they did, I saw genuine enthusiasm about moving forward in their lives.

References

Corey, M., Corey, G., & Corey, C. (2013). *Groups: Process and practice.* Boston: Cengage Learning.

Gilbert, P., & Procter, S. (2006). Compassionate mind training for people with high shame and self-criticism: Overview and pilot study of a group therapy approach. *Clinical Psychology and Psychotherapy, 13*(6), 353.

Green, Z., & Stiers, M. J. (2002). Multiculturalism and group therapy in the United States: A social constructionist perspective. *Group, 26*(3), 233–246.

Paré, D. A., Bondy, J., & Malhotra, C. (2006). Performing respect: Using enactments in group work with men who have abused. *Journal of Systemic Therapies, 25*(2), 64–79.

Yalom, I. D., & Leszcz, M. (2008). *The theory and practice of group psychotherapy.* New York: Basic Books.

8 Enlarging the Circle

Transpersonal Respect, Multiculturalism, and Social Justice

Using the model of family systems, it is possible to widen the spectrum of systems to include a global perspective. Transpersonal respect, or universal respect for greater humanity, becomes a possibility when the smaller circles of trust and respect are more deeply grounded, allowing safety to be available for further growth and expansion in a similar fashion to Maslow's hierarchy of need.

Creating ground for transpersonal or universal respect is about taking tangible respect, that for self and those close by, to incrementally larger and larger circles, such as trust in nuclear families expanding to extended families, which in turn can expand into communities, nations, and ultimately universal respect for all of humankind, such that the abstract "Other"— stranger or enemy—no longer exists in a way that poses a threat. To respect means moving past fear to embrace humanity with curiosity and confidence. Recognizing this as ideal versus the ongoing real-life situations of sometimes severely disrespectful patterns among families, communities, political factions, religions, tribes, sects, and nations, which too often lead to oppression, violent conflicts, and war, makes the case for the urgency for respect to grow.

When we consider all of the possible differences and combinations of differences there are in humanity, it can be quite overwhelming. Everything from genetics to personality traits, philosophies, beliefs, cultural mores, family backgrounds, physical and psychological attributes, as well as socio-economic and life experiences, all contribute to the vast array of differences there are between us. And yet there remains the common thread of being human. How we approach our differences is very much up to us.

Transpersonal psychology, as exemplified by the works of Ken Wilber, endeavors to study a broader framework of disciplines, philosophy, religion, science, and spirituality through the lens of psychology. It also extends the concept of identity beyond (trans) the personal—or even interpersonal— to "wider aspects of humankind"(Rothberg, Kelly, & Kelly, 1998, p. 4). It is within this line of thinking that RFT can be based within a larger framework.

Multiculturalism

The American Counseling Association Code of Ethics 2015 states, "Counselors are aware of their own values, attitudes, beliefs, and behaviors and avoid imposing values that are inconsistent with counseling goals. Counselors respect the diversity of clients, trainees, and research participants" (Section A.4.b.). The American Psychological Association (APA) and the American Association of Marriage and Family Therapists have similar such codes.

The theme of the American Association of Marriage and Family Therapists Annual Conference 2015 was multiculturalism. It is currently becoming a more prominent consideration within the psychotherapy profession and reasonably so. It has been historically lacking in our research and practice, although there was a surge in such research beginning in the 1980s and 1990s, which continues through today. I believe that we are still on the cusp of having a deeper and fuller understanding of what that means conceptually within the parameters of the work we do. The conversation around it is healthy and still badly needed.

Multiculturalism is about gaining awareness and understanding of the complexity of life experiences, be they relational, socioeconomic, or political in scope, about ethnicity, belief systems, or inherent ways of being, for example, gender, sexual orientation, or disability. It is about having tolerance and acceptance of others regardless of differences.

Williams and Levitt (2008) studied the differences between the values of therapists and clients as they relate to multiculturalism. They found substantial evidence supporting that there exist real value differences between therapists and clients and that "therapists cannot be value-neutral and that they routinely convey their values with clients." (p. 256). Therefore, they say, "[T]he potential exists for therapists to consciously or unconsciously influence clients to become more like themselves" (p. 256). They point out that most therapists are unaware of the potential negative effects of sharing such values with the client because they do so intending to benefit the client. Especially within a multicultural context, there is a higher probability of alienation, shame and/or indoctrination for the client in ways that either shut down the treatment or is counter-indicated for real progress to be gained.

The reality that therapists are not able to be value neutral by the sheer fact that we are human beings should not be a surprise. The values that we hold are not necessarily questionable, but if imposed wrongly, they create an ethical problem. This study indicates that we "routinely convey . . . consciously or unconsciously" our values to make clients become more like ourselves. From the RFT perspective, this is quite disturbing and unethical. We may not be able to monitor all that we say and do without full awareness, but if our primary focus in the therapeutic process is on the foundation of respectful interaction, then in an acutely mindful way, we need to remain curious about who our clients really are and what their values mean to them, especially as they relate to their particular culture.

I believe that intolerance is born out of fear. That is, we, as human beings, are afraid of the unfamiliar and feel somewhat threatened by the idea that unfamiliar traits may somehow negatively impact us. It is therefore in our best interest, as well as in the interest of our clients, to become as familiar and knowledgeable as possible about the wide range of human values and cultures. This is an ongoing process of growth and curiosity, one that benefits us all.

It is with this in mind that we explore various kinds of cultural differences, understanding that these differences are infinite. No two individuals will ever have exactly the same cultural footprint. But understanding some of the main areas of difference, as recognized currently in the field of multiculturalism, is vitally important. The list of designated differences that are about to be presented and discussed is in no way exhaustive but does challenge our scope of awareness, knowledge, and preconceived ideas about others.

Race, Ethnicity, and Nationality

We most frequently associate multiculturalism with ethnicity, race, and nationality. There are, of course, many ethnic groups in the world who have been oppressed historically and currently by advantaged groups predominately for economic prestige and power. The groups in the US who are most identified as " 'Visible Racial Ethnic Minority Groups' (are) African Americans, American Indians, Asian Americans and Hispanics" (Sue, Arredondo, & McDavis, 1992, p. 478). Of course, others exist such as those from the Middle East and India as well as many subcultures within larger cultures and combined ethnicities, making the possible cultural options infinite. Most significant to being a responsive, culturally sensitive therapist is the ability to understand the current cultural biases and oppression that are a present reality for each client we have sitting in our office and the others who matter to them.

African-Americans

When considering persons who identify themselves African-American, it is important to recognize that there is an abundance of research documenting the fact that the majority of African-Americans utilize mental health services much less frequently than Caucasians, indicating that many may be reluctant, if not skeptical, about the trustworthiness of mental health professionals and the value of psychotherapy in general. It is imperative to keep in mind the long and brutal history of slavery and subsequent acts of hate and subjugation this population has endured, especially in this country. Without question, this strong precedent outshines the weak attempts of many who pretend to understand. It is obvious that those of us who have never had the same collective experiences of extreme systemic humiliation and torture will never be able to completely "get it." We can only strengthen our desire to support our African-American clients by being authentically open to learning more from them about their life journeys as they understand them without our imposed, learned stereotypes. This includes the assumptions we make from an "informed" stance such as assuming that the difficulties a person is experiencing are always directly caused by racial tension.

In a study conducted by Thompson, Bazile, and Akbar (2004), through a number of focus groups of African-Americans, it was found that there are a number of factors that make this level of distrust in the mental health profession. They include the perception of stigma and weakness in asking for mental health services, from both the professionals as well as from their own community as well as the cost of services and the impersonal reception from professionals and the lack of understanding of life experiences that is different from their own, particularly as it relates to African-American culture.

Two things stood out in this study pertaining to the elements of therapy that create more acceptability to African-American clients beyond the affordability. First, it was noted that clear goals, and concrete tools and strategies for coping, as well as indications of hope for real resolution were more useful than longer-term "insight" therapy. Most importantly, the therapeutic relationship that was based on respect and understanding of their realities and them as individuals, rather than being fitted into stereotypic boxes, had significantly better outcomes.

Once again, this points to the relevance of respect as a key component in our work. Using the example of the client, Andrea, from the case study on group therapy in the last chapter, we can look at her concerns for being regarded as the "stereotypic Black girl" as it relates to her familial background. This stereotype has largely been created through the historical as well as current context of racial oppression that has systematically maintained reduction of the African-American experience, leading many to a sense of hopelessness and lowered expectations and self-worth. Andrea tried to counter these classic systems with anger and defiance. She held onto the one strength she knew she had, her intelligence, but was held back by the pressing rage inside her. Watching the destruction of her nuclear family and feeling helpless to fix it, while abandoned by them, and then having to adjust to being integrated into a different family system with an obligation of gratitude, she could not contain her sense of overwhelming injustice.

It is easy to see how a therapist could interpret this kind of internal turmoil, manifesting as external altercations, as oppositional-defiant behavior that must be stopped, lest it becomes elevated to more criminal behavior. More than anything, this projected notion of presumed criminalization needs to be replaced with a genuine concern and support for her strengths and abilities to prevail as she works through her inner conflicts and trauma. The support can be communicated both verbally and nonverbally, such that the message is clearly sent, received, and understood by the client, that the therapist is in fact open to and respectful of the realities as the client sees them. Straightforward validation of the client's unique identity is consistently necessary.

Native-Americans

Stereotyping any group of people lacks understanding and breaks the therapeutic trust necessary for real progress to be made. One prime group in the US that has historically been devastatingly misunderstood is the Native-American community. Shamefully, these original Americans were not only marginalized; they were stripped of their homelands and killed. Those who survived were banned to reservations where they no longer could freely hunt or enjoy the larger expanses of nature they worshipped. They were purposefully isolated from the new society and then later forced to assimilate into a foreign culture for their own survival. Accordingly, they had to reconfigure their value system to more align with the emerging Euro-American culture. This meant losing their sense of harmony with nature, holism, humility, anonymity, and so on to somehow be transformed into the Western values of competition, acquisition, and subjugation of nature (Heinrich, Corbine, & Thomas, 1990).

In terms of treating the mental health concerns of this population, according to these authors, the documented results have been dismal, especially among White therapists. Native-Americans, for obvious historical and cultural reasons, are typically very skeptical and suspicious of the predominately White therapists, displaying this skepticism largely through anger. The therapist then is confronted with how to respond to such anger without taking it personally. Thus, frequently there is a classic situation of transference and countertransference that results in a negative outcome for the client.

Heinrich et al. (1990) suggest that there is no one modality or technique that effectively addresses this problem. They do suggest that "the use of an existential framework that does not depend on a set of techniques but on a direct, honest dialogue focused on central, human themes" (p. 128), does have a greater potential for being successful. Additionally, they recommend learning more about culturally related metaphors, such as the vision quest, to be more relatable to the client.

Latino-Americans

This chasm of fundamental values, traditions, and ways of life between the dominate mainstream culture and the less dominate is further exemplified by the Hispanic or Latino community. This group has been officially unwelcomed into our US borders for centuries, not allowing legal status or citizenship to be as nearly available as other foreign groups, yet exploiting those who do manage to be here by expecting them to do the work no one else wants to do, for example, housekeeping, road construction, gardening, and so on. This exploitation is kept in place with the threat of deportation at any time. The manipulation for cheap labor, combined with language barriers, leaves many Hispanics and Latinos in the position of the underclass, typically in poverty and powerless to move into middle-class status.

Closely akin to the Native American experience, the mental health issues and challenges are very similar. That is, Hispanics and Latinos also are holistic and interpersonally oriented versus individualistic in principal and lifestyle (Comas-Diaz, 2006). As this researcher points out,

> Latinos' relational orientation shapes their sense of self, grounding their identity in family, ancestors, community, ethnicity, spirituality, environment, and other collective contexts. Hence, Latinos define themselves within the context of a relationship to others and to a collective.
>
> (p. 437)

Likewise, Comas-Diaz emphasizes that it is the assimilation process into a more individualistic and competitive culture, on top of the PTSD frequently acquired through the immigration process, that most creates mental health issues and the need for psychotherapy. Yet, this population, for much of the same reason, remarkably underutilizes psychotherapy. Once again, therapists need to become culturally aware of this phenomenon.

Considering the young Hispanic adolescent girl, Lucia, from the case study in the last chapter, it is obvious that she was dealing with her own assimilation issues of trying to fit in at school while also learning a new language, while at the same time, dealing with the horrific tragedy of her father's death. The family bond was so strong that Lucia and her sister risked their own safety to first find their father and then, after news of his death, to stay illegally to try to support their sick mother back home. She holds the burden of traumatic grief, being estranged from her mother and the rest of her extended family in a foreign country, trying to learn a new language and assimilate into a different culture, which is largely unwelcoming, and at the same time living in fear of deportation. For a therapist not to fully comprehend the magnitude of these burdens, with all of the nuances as they relate to mental health and treatment, is to provide deficient, if not harmful care.

Asian-Americans

Asian-Americans have a more unique position with the phenomenon of mental health alienation in that they generally are perceived to be a "model minority." That is, they often appear to not have psychological or social issues, at least at first glance (Leong & Lau, 2001). These researchers go on to point out that this larger label, "Asian," actually encompasses more than 20 separate subgroups or cultures that have distinctive characteristics and levels of resilience.

What seems to be in common for most Asians is a different sense of what medicine is, as well as what mental health or illness means in contrast to Western terms. To begin with, the Eastern medical model is much different in philosophy and protocol than Western medicine. Akin to those differences are the ways in which mental health issues are addressed. Emotional issues such as anger, grief, or depression are less recognized as a treatment-appropriate problem and more something one just handles privately. Major mental illness, that is, psychosis, which disturbs the social group, may be addressed more seriously, but Western psychotherapy might not be trusted as the desired form of treatment. The level of acculturation to the Western approaches to mental health is cited in this study as a main factor for understanding the level of engagement and acceptance. But this is also critically dependent upon the level of bias from the therapist in terms of diagnostic assessment and therapeutic intervention.

Considering the case of Cindy from the last chapter, we see a perfect example of the difficulties related to assimilation of these two cultures. She is third-generation Vietnamese-American and yet still dealing with the trust issues her parents and grandparents have handed down to her as they struggled more acutely with transitioning from their closer ties to the Eastern customs and philosophies to the foreign ways of Western tradition as well as the language barriers. Cindy has a greater opportunity and, possibly, a greater desire to become acculturated in spite of the shy reserve she has learned from her family. As we see her integrate into the group therapy dynamic, we also notice her self-confidence and respect build as she begins to feel more accepted in this environment.

On the other hand, Pam, from this case study, who is also second-generation American, but from Arab decent, is experiencing her cultural transition differently. As opposed to being reserved about her heritage, she is more angry and confused by the family dynamics, which was conflicted by the cultural differences from within that system. Her father, a first-generation Palestinian-American, had customs and beliefs from his birth country that were far more patriarchal than his American wife of blended decent was accustomed to. Hence, his need to be in charge of the family, and his wife specifically, led to his abusive behavior in reaction to her stronger Western feminine identity and the resulting split in the family. Further, his separation from his extended Palestinian family created even more personal tension for him and his relationship with his wife, a common problem among many Arab-Americans. Because this cultural perspective is more holistic, it is also more about being identified as a part of the larger familial or community system rather than an autonomous individual (Nassar McMillan & Hakim Larson, 2003).

This last point about identity, which seems to be a recurring theme among many non-Western cultures, is one that we should look at more closely as we attempt to serve these populations more effectively. In Western culture we naturally assume that autonomy is the high bar for mental health, when in fact, it really might not be for everyone. It is probably one of many embedded assumptions that we make subconsciously, which requires more focused awareness and respect. Otherwise, we risk misdiagnosis and ineffective treatment.

Differences in Religion, Faith, and Beliefs

Research on the interrelatedness of psychotherapy and religion or spirituality has been relatively sparse historically, but in the last decade or so, it has received greater interest, particularly as it relates to multiculturalism. In a study conducted by Post and Wade (2009), several interesting findings about the differences between therapists and their clients were found. First, most therapists overall were found to have significantly less personal identification with being religious or spiritual than their clients and had very little training in their counseling education around spiritual issues, yet for the most part, they saw their clients' religious beliefs or practices as a positive addition to their mental health. However, the belief systems outside of the more traditional Western religions, that is, in the Judeo-Christian tradition, were more often seen as being tied to some pathology. Eastern religions, Islam, and Native-American faiths would be typical examples of such misunderstandings.

As this study continues to point out, the pluralistic approach, that is, the broader willingness to be open to and accepting of all faiths, even those unknown to us, is perhaps the most effective and ethical stance we can have with clients. The key danger in not taking such a position is to fall into the trap described earlier of trying, consciously or subconsciously, to make clients become more like ourselves. It is not wise, particularly in therapy, to impose our beliefs on someone else, especially to those who are more vulnerable.

There are those counselors who identify themselves as Christian counselors (or other faiths), who use spiritual tools such as scripture readings and prayers within the context of doing therapy. If this is understood and agreed to by the client prior to implementing these practices, it can be a powerful tool, which may reach into the deeper spiritual needs of the client. If handled with care and respect for the client's perspective, without judgment, this can truly be an enriching process.

The religion that has come under the most scrutiny by the Western world, especially since 9/11, has been the Islamic faith. The extreme radicalization of this faith has in fact presented major devastation through violent acts of hatred and terror, which continue today by the growing militant groups in the Middle East. But the Qur'an, the Bible of the Muslim faith, teaches the values of caring for the larger community (Armstrong, 2000). Most Muslim communities are peace loving and nonviolent. Only the radical groups such as ISIS, Al Qaeda, or the Taliban, which espouse hatred, commit political violence.

Therefore, it is essential to regard persons who are Muslim with dignity and respect, unless connection to one of these groups is known. Even then, if the opportunity presents itself to be able to intervene potential violent acts in the future, such as working with a young person who is considering radicalization; without inviting harm to oneself, this is a worthy attempt to maintain a respectful posture.

Pam, from the group case study, is Muslim. She wears a hijab to school, which signals an opportunity for bullies to bully her, with adult approval. This kind of targeted hate behavior, which is passively supported, creates for her a sense of alienation and subsequent self-doubt. Additionally, in Pam's case, the split in her own family around the cultural differences between her parents further creates inner conflict and confusion of identity for her. Therapeutically, then, it becomes necessary to support her in defining her own identity, under her own terms, and assist her in strengthening her sense of self-respect in that identity, regardless of the opinions or beliefs held by the therapist. This is a difficult leap for many therapists as it may feel contradictory to one's own values, but in terms of helping clients move forward in their own paths of mental wellness, it becomes critical to be able to do just that.

Gender and Gender Identity

When considering gender differences in psychotherapy, there are multiple dynamics to reflect upon. Men and women typically process therapeutic experiences somewhat differently.

For example, men have been historically, and to some extent still are, cast by many in the mental health field as "rigidly endors(ing) emotional stoicism, competition, status, and toughness . . . (and thereby displaying traits such as) aggression and violence, homophobia, misogyny, detached fathering . . . and neglect of physical and mental health" (Englar-Carlson & Kiselica, 2013, p. 400); however, these authors suggest building a new construct of positive masculinity, which is strength based and goal oriented toward greater flexibility in identity. In their words, "Positive masculinity emphasizes the adaptive character strengths, emotions, and virtues of men that promote well-being and resiliency in self and others" (p. 401). This statement underscores the idea that by respecting men's strengths and abilities, we allow for them the opportunity to lessen the restrictions that they put upon themselves and others. In doing so, they are given the space to be able to expand their range of acceptable masculinity to include more emotional expression, vulnerability, and ability to nurture.

It has long been said that the only emotion men are allowed to express is anger, whereas the only emotion women are not allowed to express is anger. So, as restricted as men are emotionally, so are women in a very different way. Because women are much more frequently victims of abuse (physical, sexual, and psychological) than men, and because they subsequently are not able culturally to voice appropriate anger responses to such abuse and subjugation, women are more likely to internalize their anger, turning it more toward themselves than toward their abusers. As a result, women who have been abused, most specifically those who are the victims of childhood sexual abuse, tend to more readily present disorders such as "posttraumatic stress disorder, anxiety disorders, depressions, substance use disorders, eating disorders, dissociative disorders, and personality disorders" (Peleikis & Dahl, 2005, p. 304).

Women with less severe histories of abuse, but who have experienced some level of gender oppression, tend to also show signs of internalized anger, such as lowered self-respect and/or related depression. The goal of RFT, then, would be to encourage women to revalue themselves through the lens of respect and worthiness that allows for the emotion of anger expressed externally to not only be appropriate but essential in the healthy array of all emotional responses.

Persons who identify themselves as being in the LGBTQ community have long been seen, and still are, by most cultures and religions as being deviant and immoral. Until 1973, homosexuality was classified in the DSM as a mental disorder. This concept of pathologizing this community only added to the extreme prejudice, manifesting largely as hatred and cruelty, which has, until recent years, dominated the public perspective. As late as a couple of decades ago, many studies of the LBGTQ population in the mental health field were still focused on trying to "cure" homosexuality by "making them straight," even as it was becoming more and more empirically evident that homosexuality is not a disease or a disorder or even a choice but a way of being. Studies in the 1980s and 1990s focused on biological-oriented differences based in genetic, brain, and hormonal factors to be definitive answers to the cause of homosexuality, but many of these studies were later found to be flawed because they failed to incorporate bisexuality and transgendered persons, thus not considering other factors such as culture and sociopsychological implications (Parker, 2014). Though the exact "cause" of may not be defined conclusively, the reality is that persons in this community are not somehow defected, needing to be "fixed."

Semlyen, Killaspy, Nazareth, and Osborn (2007) reviewed studies related to the acceptability and efficacy of counseling approaches with the LGBTQ community. As with other nondominant populations, once again, the results of various studies concluded that what made therapy most successful was the element of clients feeling safe and not judged by the therapist. Many LGBTQ clients, especially those who have not yet fully come to a stronger identity within themselves about their sexuality, are more likely to seek therapists who have like sexual orientations, primarily because of the fear of awkward misunderstandings and having to educate the therapists who have probing, unrelated questions about their lifestyles, if not blatant, expressed prejudices. This requires that the therapist is knowledgeable and comfortable with this community, such that the therapy is affirming of the various lifestyles, be it gay, lesbian, bisexual, and/or transgender. The more welcoming the therapist is of the client, communicating ease and awareness about various sexual practices without pathologizing or condemning them, the more willing and able the client is to be engaged, benefitting greater from this experience.

The case presented in the fifth chapter of this book was about a gay couple, Will and Troy, who loved one another very much but were having trouble. Will was coming from a heterosexual marriage and was a devout Baptist Christian, who for most of his life believed that homosexuality was perhaps the worst sin one could ever commit. But he could not any longer deny the feelings he had always had for men, especially since he had met Troy, whom he had fallen madly in love with.

Troy, who had been out for all of his sexually active life and was very settled with his identity, was troubled by Will's past with such traditional values and beliefs. He, however, had not before been in a committed relationship as long or as serious as this one and therefore brought many of his own anxieties into this relationship.

My job was to first establish their trust and confidence in me as a competent, well-informed therapist on LBGTQ issues who showed each man fair, respectful concern for who they were in their sexuality but also in their totality as human beings. Beyond that, I was to be the guide and the catalyst to aid them in finding their own sense of honor in who they both were individually and who they could become as a couple. This encompassed helping Will integrate his sense of faith and family values with his newfound identity, without shame, but rather as a complete person with integrity and dignity. Likewise, Troy, who was more secure in his sexual identity, lacked security in his attachments in relationships and needed assistance in learning how to allow himself the vulnerability to truly bond with someone in genuine love. As a couple, they needed to learn how to move past their fears so that they could honor one another more deeply. As their therapist, I was immensely honored to be part of that process.

Persons With Disabilities

Persons with disabilities, within the study of multiculturalism, have been, until recent years, relatively disregarded as a seriously marginalized subgroup to be examined. Much of the difficulty in identifying this group is that it is not homogeneous. There is such a wide range of different types of disabilities—intellectual, psychiatric and physical—each containing many variant kinds of challenges per individual. These can range from, for example, severe intellectual challenges to an array of learning disabilities, schizophrenia to the autism spectrum, blindness, deafness, and motor and/ or mobility impairment.

Additionally, persons with disabilities tend to not self-identify with other kinds of disabilities; for example, mobility-impaired persons don't typically identify with persons on the autism spectrum or those who are intellectually challenged, and blind or deaf individuals typically don't identify with the mobility impaired. This creates splintering among the larger umbrella of disability, making it seem like smaller pockets of the population and therefore not an identifiable minority. However, collectively, it is the largest minority group in the world.

What unifies this group, unfortunately, is the cluster of similar responses persons with disabilities typically receive from the nondisabled population. Such responses often include ignoring, talking down to, avoiding, bullying, abusing, and so on. As a person with a motor/mobility impairment, cerebral palsy, I am acutely aware of these responses, as I have encountered them in different contexts and degrees all of my life.

What I am equally aware of, as I mature, is that most, if not all, of these responses are based in fear of the unknown and, at a deeper level, fear of experiencing one's own limitations in a more pronounced way. However the affected realities for the person who receives those responses can, in fact, be demoralizing if not devastating. RFT requires us, as clinicians, to be aware of and sensitive to the ways in which our internal responses to different disabilities may be consciously or subconsciously impacting our work. Learning more about various disabilities, as well as checking our own emotional responses, is highly recommended.

Cindy from the group therapy case study, for example, had a cleft pallet, which was physically disfiguring to her face as well as creating some speech issues for her. Her lack of language command combined with her speech impediment led to being laughed at and bullied at school. Her therapist needs to be fully aware of this probability, even if the client, especially a child or adolescent client, doesn't mention it. Again, therapists also need to be noticing their own responses of discomfort so as to not add to the sense of unacceptability.

Ageism

Ageism is a closely related issue when dealing with seniors, especially those with related cognitive impairments, such as Alzheimer's and dementia. As people age, at some point or in gradated degrees, certain abilities decline, including sight, hearing, strength, and so on.

Often therapists feel as though there is little to no benefit that can result from therapy with impaired seniors because they are unable to comprehend or have insufficient insight to be able to process effectively. Nelson (2005) suggests that mental health professionals, as well as other health providers, for example, physicians, tend to practice with "professional ageism" or "healthism"—that pervasive heath issues make treatment seem more futile and less valuable. He suggests further that most health professionals, mental health included, are implicitly trained to hold such biases such that younger patients or clients are regarded to be more important than their older counterparts, who are expected to have worse prognoses and outcomes. This author goes on to promote the need for more intentional, proactive education for all health professionals toward better care of the aging client. Psychotherapists need to once again become aware of their own fears of aging and related biases, avoiding pitfalls such as overcompensated language or having lowered or devalued expectations for the aging client.

Poverty

The common denominator of most of the marginalized groups mentioned is, unfortunately, poverty or lowered socioeconomic status. Therefore, access to mental health services is diminished even further largely due to a lack of resources. Santiago, Kaltman, and Miranda (2013) point out that the lower-income population has a disproportionately higher need for mental health services because of the heavier stresses that accompany poverty, trying to meet just basic needs—food, a place to stay, care for family, and so on—as well as all the relational conflicts that can occur as a result as consequences to that strain. PTSD is more prevalent in this population, largely due to more conflict and violence, which are outgrowths of the struggles caused by poverty. Children as well as adults are victims of this environment emotionally and psychologically. Yet, as these same authors note, there is significant research supporting the fact that these same individuals can and do respond just as favorably to mental health services as other populations more privileged, when given the opportunity. Finally, this study suggests that whereas lack of financial resources is a primary barrier for lower-income people to receive mental health services, there are other, deeper barriers including attitudinal and larger systemic issues that help ensure the financial barriers remain in place and that mental health services are minimally provided.

Smith (2005) regards this as classism, which she defines as "a form of oppression . . . an interlocking system that involves domination and control of social ideology, institutions and resources" (p. 688). She goes further to explore the decades historically back as far as the 1940s to examine the ways in which classism was presented and responded to within the mental health field. Essentially, she finds that whereas attempts have been made to address this problem, including an APA Resolution in 2000, which said, " 'poverty is detrimental to psychological well-being" and charged psychologists with the responsibility to 'treat and address the needs of low-income individuals and families' " (p. 690), not much progress on this endemic problem has been made to present.

Social Justice

In conjunction with the inequities outlined throughout this chapter, related to minority and oppressed cultural or social status, Constantine, Hage, Kindaichi, and Bryant (2007), discuss the importance of social justice and the constructive, proactive role counselors and therapists can and should take in therapy. They explain, "Social justice reflects a fundamental valuing of fairness and equity in resources, rights, and treatment for marginalized individuals and groups of people" (p. 24). They go on further to explain how the therapist implements social justice by fulfilling several different roles inside and outside of the therapeutic office: "The roles of adviser, consultant, advocate, and change agent embody tenets of social justice and activism through client empowerment and advocacy."

Lee (2007) states emphatically that it is a counselor's duty to advocate for social justice.

> In the counseling context, social justice encompasses the professional, ethical, and moral responsibility that counselors have to address the social, cultural and economic inequalities that may negatively affect the psychosocial development of various groups of people. Social justice relates to counselors' sense of social responsibility.
>
> (p. vii)

It is with this imperative that RFT stands. To be fully respectful of all human beings means more than just being polite and courteous to those who enter the therapy room. It requires bold intention to act toward the betterment of humanity as a whole. It means shining a light on each person's dignity and giving that dignity the psychosocial space to grow.

So, what does this mean to advocate for clients in practical terms? It could begin to be as simple as offering a sliding scale or reduced fees so that lower-income persons have the welcomed opportunity to get therapy at all. Beyond this initial entry, it is about empowerment for the client's ability to self-advocate for rights denied by family, friends, employers, landlords, schools, and so on, giving him or her tools but also, and more importantly, fostering the confidence necessary to continue self-advocacy in the future. Realistically, it often means that we, as fellow human beings, take a larger role in direct advocacy by speaking on behalf of our clients to schools, doctors, agencies, parole or probation officers, and so on. Indirectly, our broader sense of social justice advocacy, may include our roles on nonprofit boards or political involvement for legislative or policy changes that enhance the civil rights for our clients and other disenfranchised groups, which extend throughout the world.

As we start to consider the work we are engaged in from a macro perspective, we can begin to imagine how the influence of RFT might start to shift more universal paradigms. As intrapersonal conflicts are resolved through gaining more respect for oneself and affects the interpersonal relationships that person has, those relationships affect systems, which are a part of larger systems, becoming global in dimension.

Looking at the world as it is now, with the phenomenon of terrorist activity, which stems from such a deep disrespect for opposing religious views, political and territorial conflicts arise into violent and horrific outcomes. It becomes easy to blame one side over another when we see such destruction happening by the actions demonstrated by that particular side. Throughout recorded time there has always been an "Other" to be hated and defeated (Rowlett, 1996). This isn't to diminish the level of atrocities that one side commits, for example, Hitler's Holocaust or Isis's and al Qaeda's attacks throughout the world, but to emphasize the ongoing, repetitive nature of such occurrences. For most of us, this feels endlessly defeating, that this state of war and human division is a permanent condition in our existence.

It may be a foolish, naïve proposition to make, but what if a genuine, deeply rooted, deeply felt, and strongly acted upon sense of respect could permeate our entire atmosphere in all directions? This is pie-in-the-sky thinking to be sure. But what if Buber's I-It model of human interaction could slowly, deliberately, be replaced with his concept of the I-Thou? What if, we as therapists could, both individually and collectively worldwide, start creating such a shift by authentically practicing RFT?

References

American Counseling Association (2014). *ACA Code of Ethics*. Alexandria, VA: Author.

Armstrong, Karen. (2000). *Islam: A short history*. New York: Modern Library.

Comas-Diaz, L. (2006). Latino healing: The integration of ethnic psychology into psychotherapy. *Psychotherapy: Theory, Research, Practice, Training, 43*(4), 436.

Constantine, M. G., Hage, S. M., Kindaichi, M. M., & Bryant, R. M. (2007). Social justice and multicultural issues: Implications for the practice and training of counselors and counseling psychologists. *Journal of Counseling & Development, 85*(1), 24.

Englar-Carlson, M., & Kiselica, M. S. (2013). Affirming the strengths in men: A positive masculinity approach to assisting male clients. *Journal of Counseling & Development, 91*(4), 399–409.

Heinrich, R. K., Corbine, J. L., & Thomas, K. R. (1990). Counseling Native Americans. *Journal of Counseling & Development, 69*(2), 128–133.

Lee, C. C. (2007). *Counseling for social justice*. Alexandria, VA: American Counseling Association.

Leong, F. T., & Lau, A. S. (2001). Barriers to providing effective mental health services to Asian Americans. *Mental Health Services Research, 3*(4), 201–214.

Nassar-McMillan, S. C., & Hakim-Larson, J. (2003). Counseling considerations among Arab Americans. *Journal of Counseling & Development, 81*(2), 150–159.

Nelson, T. D. (2005). Ageism: Prejudice against our feared future self. *Journal of Social Issues, 61*(2), 207–221.

Parker, D. A. (2014). *Sex, cells, and same-sex desire: The biology of sexual preference*. New York: Routledge.

Peleikis, D. E., & Dahl, A. A. (2005). A systematic review of empirical studies of psychotherapy with women who were sexually abused as children. *Psychotherapy Research, 15*(3), 304–315.

Post, B. C., & Wade, N. G. (2009). Religion and spirituality in psychotherapy: A practice-friendly review of research. *Journal of Clinical Psychology, 65*(2), 131–146.

Rothberg, D. J., Kelly, S. M., & Kelly, S. (Eds.). (1998). *Ken Wilber in dialogue: Conversations with leading transpersonal thinkers.* Wheaton, IL: Quest Books.

Rowlett, L. L. (1996). *Joshua and the rhetoric of violence: A new historicist analysis.* Sheffield, UK: Sheffield Academic Press, Ltd.

Santiago, C. D., Kaltman, S., & Miranda, J. (2013). Poverty and mental health: How do low-income adults and children fare in psychotherapy? *Journal of Clinical Psychology, 69*(2), 115–126.

Semlyen, J., Killaspy, H., Nazareth, I., & Osborn, D. (2007). A Systematic Review of Research on Counselling and Psychotherapy for Lesbian, Gay, Bisexual & Transgender People. London: British Association for Counseling and Psychotherapy.

Smith, L. (2005). Psychotherapy, classism, and the poor: Conspicuous by their absence. *American Psychologist, 60*(7), 687.

Sue, Arredondo and McDavis, (1992), Multicultural counseling competencies and standards: a call to the profession. *Journal of Counseling & Development*, 70(4) 477–486.

Thompson, V. L. S., Bazile, A., & Akbar, M. (2004). African Americans' perceptions of psychotherapy and psychotherapists. *Professional Psychology: Research and Practice, 35*(1), 19.

Williams, D., & Levitt, H. M. (2008). Clients' experiences of difference with therapists: Sustaining faith in psychotherapy. *Psychotherapy Research, 18*(3), 256–270.

9 Therapist Respect Thyself
Maintaining Balance and Self-Care

For therapists to be able to do this work with clarity and professional longitude, it must be clear that we have to be able to maintain a high degree of respect for ourselves as well as for others. As we immerse ourselves in the business of attending to the needs of others, as with any helping profession, taking care of our own needs and physical, spiritual, and emotional well-being is vitally important. Having a solid sense of self, with good boundaries and yet a good heart, is what makes us most valuable to others. How can we ask our clients to honor themselves if we aren't doing it ourselves?

Beyond that, it becomes an ethical issue, parallel to respecting our clients; we must also respect ourselves and our human capacities to hold the pain and confusion our clients bring to us. If we are to honor those painful experiences of our clients as well as who they are in their unique humanity, including those who we might privately disagree with in terms of choices and values that are theirs, then where is there room for our own perspectives and feelings? How can we identify and maintain our beliefs, thoughts, feelings, and perspectives if we are called to be so "Other" focused? The answers are not simple; they require the ability for serious introspection. They require a sense of self-knowledge and balance from within.

Burnout and Clinical Impairment

Burnout is something that we all dread but is also something that most of us assume will never happen to us. Barnett, Baker, Elman, and Schoener (2007) say that burnout is "the terminal phase of therapist distress." They go further to describe:

> It is characterized by feelings of depersonalization, emotional exhaustion, and a lack of feelings of satisfaction and accomplishment, and it may result from prolonged work with emotionally challenging clients. Similarly, clinical work with victims of violence and other traumatic events may lead to vicarious traumatization, or secondary victimization.
>
> (p. 604)

Burnout left unchecked, then, can lead to clinical impairment. The national mental health professional organizations, such as the APA, American Counseling Association, American Association of Marriage and Family Therapists, and National Association of Social Workers address in their codes of ethics the issue of clinical impairment. They unanimously agree that it is unethical for impaired clinicians to practice, such that the impairment might be harmful to the clients served, although none of these organizations definitively specify the parameters of impairment. For example, the APA code standard on this issue states:

2.06 Personal Problems and Conflicts

(a) Psychologists refrain from initiating an activity when they know or should know that there is a substantial likelihood that their personal problems will prevent them from performing their work-related activities in a competent manner.

(b) When psychologists become aware of personal problems that may interfere with their performing work-related duties adequately, they take appropriate measures, such as obtaining professional consultation or assistance and determine whether they should limit, suspend or terminate their work-related duties.

The difficulty with this and other similar codes is that there is no clear definition or delineation of what impairment is or how one determines what level of impairment mandates termination, other than when it causes harm to clients. This, too, is subjective and falls mainly to the individual practitioner, a peer or group of peers, or results from a board review action in response to a complaint or lawsuit brought by a client. Therefore, the practitioner must address and manage any signs of ongoing distress, preferably preventing them with good self-care.

Self-Care

The means by which we manage to avoid burnout and possible psychological impairment is varied as each individual has different needs and strengths. Self-care is, however, the umbrella over each set of strategies that we might employ and is critical to maintain our well-being as competent clinicians.

Richards, Campenni, and Muse-Burke (2010) offer that there are three primary areas of self-care that need our attention for overall wellness. First, our physical needs for activity, rest, and relaxation, as well as good nutritional eating habits, are the most basic, fundamental requirements we all need to carefully attend to routinely. Being in caregiver roles, it is easy to lose that attention with our time being focused on appointments, paperwork, meetings, and so on. More significantly, many of us tend to immerse ourselves in our work directly with clients to such an extent that we lose focus on our own basic needs. This reality can be true for other health-care professions as well, but the unique feature for those in mental health is the degree to which we become intimately involved with each of our clients' lives and that takes a special sort energy that involves our emotional resources as well as cognitive abilities.

Second, and perhaps the most profound area for therapists to be diligently aware of, is our own psychological wellness. Richards et al. (2010) note that a great many of us who go into psychotherapy as a profession come from dysfunctional family backgrounds and have experienced some form of abuse and/or familial substance abuse or mental illness. This experiential background often motivates many of us to go into this field and also creates a higher susceptibility to being emotionally triggered by the traumatic content shared with us by our clients. Even for those who do not have such backgrounds, handling the information we receive day after day can still take a toll on us mentally and emotionally. Therefore it is frequently suggested that therapists seek their own therapy as a professional safety valve to prevent overload and burnout.

There are additional means of countering the kind of emotional distress that can contribute to burnout or compassion fatigue (Figley, 2002). Balance in our personal and professional lives is perhaps one of the most obvious but often not so easy to achieve. Having our own social and interpersonal support network is critical for us to have anchored footing from which we can recharge. Whatever that support looks like, be it significant others, family, friends, or colleagues, it needs to be sustaining and provide safety for us as we realign ourselves with our own set of realities. Being able to engage with others in such a way that is mutually beneficial is imperative for us to maintain our balance.

Attuning to our spiritual needs is the third area of self-care. This can be interpreted in a multitude of ways. Spirituality is a highly personal thing, even within the same religion or outside of religion all together. The researchers mentioned here suggest that the data supports the idea that spiritual connection of some form generally contributes to personal purpose and meaning. This addresses our inner core values and that which we hold to be precious within ourselves as well as whatever God or deity we may or may not believe in.

Mindfulness and self-awareness are related key components in our arsenal of self-care (Shaprio, Brown and Biegel, 2007). Mindfulness is about being aware of the present experience. What is currently around us externally, in our environment, and how are we responding to it? Is it inviting and pleasant to us, or is it disturbing us, and what if anything can we do to make it more comfortable? Internally, in the moment, what is our mood, our state of being?

Self-awareness, on the other hand, is more complete in the sense that it is an ongoing, evolving process that assesses at a deeper level what our needs and values are and how well we are attending to them. This evaluative process requires therapists to tune in regularly to our states of being. It also requires us to use our ability to be respectful of what it is we are tuning into. If we notice, for example, that we are becoming more and more bored, depressed, or anxious with our work, we may want to look deeper into what needs in our personal lives are not getting met. Norcross (2000) calls this "counterconditioning," or taking the necessary action, which we do for our own best interest.

Not only do we need to know how to maintain a status quo baseline of being OK but also to learn how to meet our needs in a nourishing way, allowing for personal growth to continue. Just like our clients, we cannot afford to stagnate; we are ever-evolving creatures, growing into our own maturity and wisdom.

Interpersonally, we have a need for intimacy or closeness with others in a way that is satisfying our needs as well as those of other person. Our client relationships mandate that we do not seek to serve our personal needs in this regard, but we run the risk of overlapping our needs into theirs if we are lacking our sense of meaningful connection in other places. Thus, the value of continuously investing the time and energy into the quality of our relationships with significant others, family, and friends is a vital piece of taking care of ourselves. Allowing ourselves to pay attention to those we love and those who love us, and actively cultivating those relationships into stronger, healthier bonds, frees us to be more available and selflessly present with our clients.

Beyond the interpersonal is the intrapersonal sense of well-being, which can and should expand consistently as we grow into our humanness. Again, our potential for growth is ongoing and needs not to be stymied in any way. Our exploration for greater knowledge and creative expression outside of our therapy world is just as valuable as what we gain professionally. Finding interests in different avenues like painting, music, photography, or gardening helps us develop and maintain greater balance in our lives. Using different parts of our brain for varied activities gives us the opportunity to replenish our interest in our work. Similarly, as Norcross (2000) notes, mixing up the kinds of work we do, for example, seeing individuals as well as families or teaching and supervising as well as seeing clients, can serve in keeping the content of our work fresh and stimulating.

Quiet contemplation and reflection can provide a space for therapists to consider how to better respect the flawed but whole persons we really are. Taking the time to remind ourselves of our strengths and values, thereby validating our human existence, is central to our ability to continue helping others do the same.

Therefore, many of the same tools we offer to our clients for building and maintaining self-respect are useful to us as well. For example, journaling, writing affirmations, setting personal goals, and remaining cognizant of our own beliefs and values are instrumental in holding onto a solid foundation from which we can operate effectively with and for others.

Counseling Education and Supervision

Finally, I want to include a word about counselor education and supervision. As a clinical supervisor, I have observed that counseling students and interns often feel insecure about their abilities to be good therapists. Much of this insecurity has to do primarily with their lack of experience and recedes as they grow more familiar with the hands-on process of therapy. But some of that insecurity appears to be linked to not feeling fully supported by their academic departments or previous supervisors. Some have gone so far as to say outright that they have felt chastised, even bullied by their faculty, supervisors, and/or peers.

Ramos-Sánchez et al. (2002) conducted a national survey study of negative supervisory experiences for supervisees. In the category of interpersonal conflicts between supervisors and supervisees, they cite this example:

> I feel my current supervisor is very unclear and inconsistent with her expectations of me. I feel she does not give constructive feedback but is generally critical and not conscious of how her way of delivering supervision impacts my therapy and confidence.
>
> (p. 200)

They follow this and other examples of their overall results with this statement: "These findings suggest that the impact of a negative supervisory experience is global and long lasting, causing supervisees to question their choice of career and possibly change their career plans" (p. 200). In other words, support for students or interns to respect themselves or have self-care skills seems to be lacking within the learning environment for many of these students. Whereas assessments need to be made about clinical skills and to some extent personality qualities and mental health, it seems that supportive encouragement needs to parallel what we are asking of these budding professionals to provide: support for their clients.

Barnett and Cooper (2009) discuss the ongoing, as well as acute, need for graduate programs to incorporate trainings in self-care. As they point out, "For graduate students, a culture of self-care must be established immediately. . . . Graduate programs must offer students ongoing presentations on these topics, such as through formal coursework and regularly scheduled colloquia" (p. 18). Helping students and interns develop the skills and perspective of self-care as a necessary component of our ability to do good therapy, as well as being mentally healthy individuals, is vitally important to the education process. The more we can encourage new therapists to build a solid foundation for themselves early in their careers, the greater chance they have for sustaining a truly successful and meaningful practice.

If we are to respect our clients completely as fellow human beings, we must also be able to create that same experience of full, unconditional respect toward ourselves. This does not mean that we have the illusion of perfection, but goodness can exist within us, with full expectation that there is always opportunity to grow. This is what gives us a basis for a stronger, more healing connection with clients.

References

APA Code of Ethics

Barnett, J. E., Baker, E. K., Elman, N. S., & Schoener, G. R. (2007). In pursuit of wellness: The self-care imperative. *Professional Psychology: Research and Practice, 38*(6), 603a.

Barnett, J. E., & Cooper, N. (2009). Creating a culture of self-care. *Clinical Psychology: Science and Practice, 16*(1), 16–20.

Figley, C. R. (2002). Compassion fatigue: Psychotherapists' chronic lack of self care. *Journal of Clinical Psychology, 58*(11), 1433–1441.

Norcross, J. C. (2000). Psychotherapist self-care: Practitioner-tested, research-informed strategies. *Professional Psychology: Research and Practice, 31*(6), 710.

Ramos-Sánchez, L., Esnil, E., Goodwin, A., Riggs, S., Touster, L. O., Wright, L. K., . . . & Rodolfa, E. (2002). Negative supervisory events: Effects on supervision and supervisory alliance. *Professional Psychology: Research and Practice, 33*(2), 197.

Richards, K., Campenni, C., & Muse-Burke, J. (2010). Self-care and well-being in mental health professionals: The mediating effects of self-awareness and mindfulness. *Journal of Mental Health Counseling, 32*(3), 247–264.

Shapiro, S. L., Brown, K. W., & Biegel, G. M. (2007). Teaching self-care to caregivers: Effects of mindfulness-based stress reduction on the mental health of therapists in training. *Training and Education in Professional Psychology, 1*(2), 105.

Conclusion

RFT is an approach to psychotherapy that embraces and supplements all modalities, theoretical approaches, and techniques by concentrating on the operative meaning and healing power of respect. In doing so, we custom-fit theoretical modalities and tools around the particular needs of every individual, couple, or family, while we work to help them expand their personal and interpersonal experiences in a genuinely respectful way. It is with full intention and focus on respect in the therapeutic relationship and process that RFT operates.

The root of the word respect, *respectare* or *respicere*, means literally "to look back," or to reconsider, which becomes a powerful asset in the therapeutic relationship and process. The therapeutic relationship is central toward developing an environment in which the process can expand or create more respectful experiences for the client. It is in this relationship that we have the most unique opportunity to intersect in our clients' lives, showing them what respect can really be and feel like. The underlying hypothesis of RFT is that being genuinely respected, having a taste of what Buber calls the I-Thou experience, makes it more possible to respect oneself as well as others. So we, as therapists, have a profound responsibility to put in place that needed healing component as the top priority.

The process of RFT follows this focused relationship in a way that allows the client to not only experience respect but to become more aware of it emotionally and cognitively. Internalizing this awareness in such a way that it shifts the client's perspectives and actions to become more positive and functional is the ultimate goal of RFT.

The first step in this process is, for the therapist, to fully honor the power of the pain the client is holding, such that he or she can feel honored and begin to honor the pain also. Doing so changes the way in which that pain is carried. This part of the process is similar to empathy but goes a stretch further by incorporating a different way of thinking about it. The pain, most frequently, is centered on trauma, which often carries with it some shame, complicating the level of injury done. In honoring or respecting the pain and the emotions around it, it becomes a little easier for the client to begin externalizing and separating one's identity from that pain.

At this point, especially when working with individuals, it is possible to help the client start to rebuild, or perhaps build for the first time, a sense of genuine self-respect. Again, respect is inclusive of esteem, yet goes deeper. Respect for oneself definitely includes affirmations of one's talents and strengths but also a richer appreciation for one's core values, dignity and integrity, and spirituality (for those who identify themselves as being spiritual).

A large part of this internal reevaluation, or "looking again," is dependent upon some form of self-forgiveness, which cannot be forced but rather allowed to happen. Similarly, this becomes a critical truth when working with relational issues.

Couples therapy demonstrates this truth routinely. The addition of relationship concerns to those of each individual brings further complexity to the therapeutic process. Not only are there now injuries belonging to two individuals, but there is also damage being done to and from each person, creating injury to the relationship. The disrespect often is in the form of abuse or betrayal. Establishing a stronger base of respect for each person and, therefore, the relationship, requires building support and safety between the two, something they may have never experienced in their families of origin. In doing so, trust and true intimacy have a chance to repair and grow.

The work of family therapy again increases complexity, not just because of the added number of people in the room but also the additional numbers of relational configurations, dyads, and triads as well as the generational layers of learned behavior. The construct of respect is developmental; that is, it is learned in stages throughout childhood, adolescence, and adulthood. That means if parental figures are not able to teach such behavior and attitudes through modeling, allowing the child to first experience respect for him- or herself, then that development will naturally be delayed or halted from lack of familiarity. This does not preclude correction of misguided behavior; it does suggest, however, that safety, support, and trust must be in the foundation of the family unit for respectful development to take place in a meaningful way.

When working with groups, the dynamics shift somewhat because, typically, there is no prior relationship between the members of that group. They initially come in as strangers, seemingly with no common background, except for, perhaps, the assigned topic of the group, for example, adolescent girls with troubled backgrounds or men with aggressive or anger issues. At first there is no basis for trust, much less, respect. The process of building group cohesion by facilitating the bonding of strangers, moving insecure attachments into healthier, more secure attachments, can parallel a family system in a way that introduces, as Yalom says, hope, altruism, and interpersonal learning. If done well, it can also increase self-compassion and respect for a larger world.

Finally, and perhaps most importantly, is the matter of universal respect. That means, simply, a broader sense of global respect for humanity, or transpersonal respect. We owe it to our clients to be as culturally unbiased and informed as possible so that our ability to respect others can extend beyond any barriers, be they geographical, ethnic, faith, gender, age, or ability related. Research shows that therapists tend to, knowingly or not, try to make their clients become more like themselves in terms of thought, perspective, belief, emotion, and action. This is the antithesis of what RFT is about. We are to move back our judgments and personal values to clear space for those that match what is good and right for our clients, not for ourselves.

Where, then, is the space for us, for our needs, thoughts, beliefs, and emotions? It's not in our therapy room with our clients, but it must have the top shelf in our private lives. We are duty bound to respect and care for ourselves as much as we do anyone else. It is essential that we care for ourselves physically, emotionally, psychologically, and spiritually so that we can optimally be available to give the total respect that each one of our clients deserves.

In this world, at this moment, and throughout history, there has been conflict, division, hatred, and pain. There is war, atrocity, and terror beyond our imagination. Individual lives are shattered daily by abuses of all kinds, and these people experience loss and the lack of feeling loved and accepted for exactly who they are, as they are. Therapists have the rare privilege to provide opportunities for meaningful change. We can do so most effectively by interjecting the simple antidote to most human suffering: unvarnished and true respect.

Index